# THE EAT-CLEAN DIET

## *Workout Journal*

Published by Robert Kennedy Publishing
5775 McLaughlin Road
Mississauga, ON
L5R 3P7 Canada
Visit us at **www.eatcleandiet.com**
and **www.toscareno.com**

Design by Gabriella Caruso Marques
Edited by Wendy Morley and Rachel Corradetti

National Library of Canada Cataloguing in Publication

Reno, Tosca, 1959-
        The Eat-Clean Diet Workout Journal / Tosca Reno.

ISBN-13: 978-1-55210-049-3
ISBN-10: 1-55210-049-9


        1. Physical fitness for women.  2. Stretching exercises.  3. Cardiovascular fitness.
    4. Weight training for women. I. Title.

RA781.6.R462 2008                613.7'045                C2007-906808-1


10 9 8 7 6 5 4 3 2


Distributed in Canada by
NBN (National Book Network)
67 Mowat Avenue, Suite 241
Toronto, ON
M6K 3E3

Distributed in USA by
NBN (National Book Network)
15200 NBN Way
Blue Ridge Summit, PA
17214

Printed in Canada

## IMPORTANT

The information in this book reflects the author's experiences and opinions and is not intended to replace medical advice.

Before beginning this or any nutritional or exercise regimen, consult your physician to be sure it is appropriate for you. Ask for a physical stress test.

# GENERAL INFORMATION

NAME _____

ADDRESS _____

CITY _____ STATE _____ ZIP _____

PHONE _____

FAX _____

COMPANY NAME _____

ADDRESS _____

CITY _____ STATE _____ ZIP _____

PHONE _____

FAX _____

# EMERGENCY INFORMATION

NOTIFY _____ RELATIONSHIP _____

PHONE _____ WORK PHONE _____

ADDRESS _____

CITY _____ STATE _____ ZIP _____


OR NOTIFY _____ RELATIONSHIP _____

PHONE _____ WORK PHONE _____

ADDRESS _____ STATE _____ ZIP _____

# MEDICAL INFORMATION

PHYSICIAN _____ PHONE _____

INSURANCE/HMO _____

BLOOD TYPE _____ ALLERGIES _____

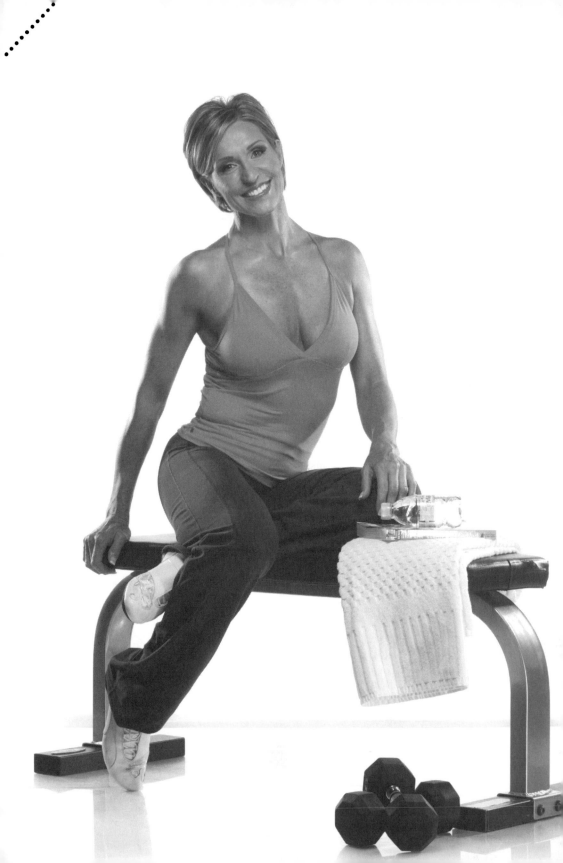

# EAT CLEAN FOR HEALTH AND FOR LIFE

**I** always stress the importance of recording your progress. Virtually every other weight-loss program stresses the same thing. How do you know where you are going if you don't know where you have been? You need to put pen to paper and write down your triumphs and yes, even your defeats, as you become a Sister in Iron. Somehow the act of recording little details about your workouts brings a sense of accountability to the process. If I work out and don't write it down it's as if I have not even done that session. Sometimes when I travel I forget to bring along my journal. With no record of what I have done I don't know what body part I trained, how many sets and reps, or how I was feeling that day. So write it down!

My training journal is just the tool for the job. This little book will become your fast friend in the gym. Keep it handy while you do the good work: the weight training, the cardio, the sweating, the motivation. The journal becomes the story of YOU. This will become a very good story. Commit to recording the little details of your journey as you build the best YOU possible. Since it is filled with my training tips and inspiration, I hope you feel as if this record brings me a little closer to you.

Remember, I am always listening.

Sincerely,

Tosca Reno

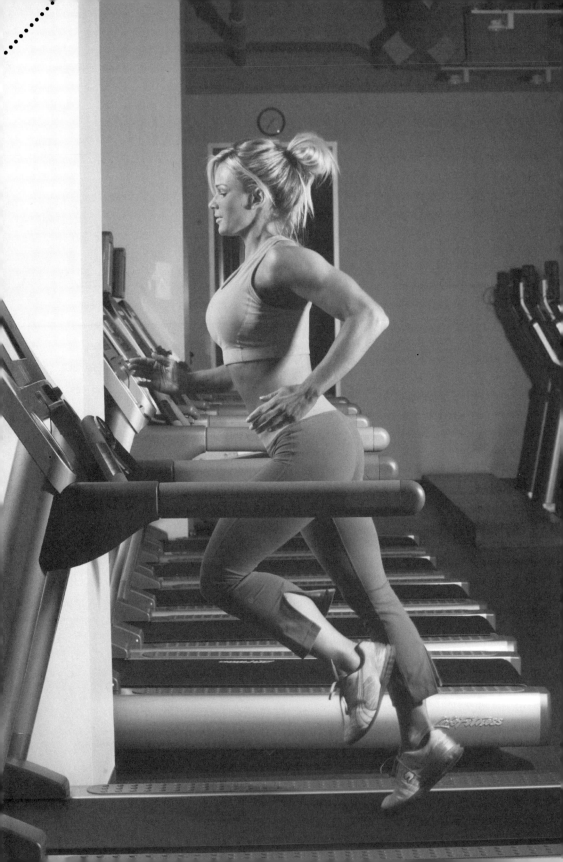

# CALCULATING INTENSITY LEVELS

Your heart rate is a good indicator of your intensity level during your cardio workouts. If it is between 55 and 80 percent of your maximum heart rate, or MHR, then you are training aerobically. This means "with oxygen," and is an activity that can be carried out for long periods of time. If your heart rate is between 80 and 100 percent of your MHR, then you are training anaerobically. You will be able to train this way for short bursts, but not for extended periods.

Cardio training should be done for a minimum of 20 minutes at a time. You can go steadily and stay in a given heart-rate zone, or you can do interval training, in which case you work in both the aerobic and anaerobic zones. Interval training is by far the most effective for improving cardiovascular fitness and for burning calories, but this is an intensity technique and you'll have to work your way up to it! Be sure to visit your doctor for a stress test before beginning any exercise program.

**To figure out your maximum heart rate, subtract your age from 220. Multiply by 0.55, 0.65, 0.75 and 0.85 to determine your optimal heart-rate training ranges.**

• **Beginners** should should stay between 55 and 65 percent of their MHR.

• **Intermediates** can work in the range of 65 to 75 percent.

• **Advanced** trainers can work steadily in the 75-to-85-percent range, and can go even higher for short bursts, if they're in good enough condition.

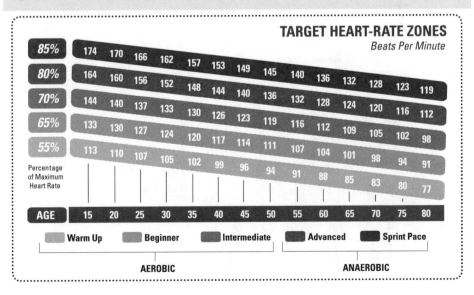

### TARGET HEART-RATE ZONES
*Beats Per Minute*

| | 15 | 20 | 25 | 30 | 35 | 40 | 45 | 50 | 55 | 60 | 65 | 70 | 75 | 80 |
|---|---|---|---|---|---|---|---|---|---|---|---|---|---|---|
| **85%** | 174 | 170 | 166 | 162 | 157 | 153 | 149 | 145 | 140 | 136 | 132 | 128 | 123 | 119 |
| **80%** | 164 | 160 | 156 | 152 | 148 | 144 | 140 | 136 | 132 | 128 | 124 | 120 | 116 | 112 |
| **70%** | 144 | 140 | 137 | 133 | 130 | 126 | 123 | 119 | 116 | 112 | 109 | 105 | 102 | 98 |
| **65%** | 133 | 130 | 127 | 124 | 120 | 117 | 114 | 111 | 107 | 104 | 101 | 98 | 94 | 91 |
| **55%** | 113 | 110 | 107 | 105 | 102 | 99 | 96 | 94 | 91 | 88 | 85 | 83 | 80 | 77 |

Percentage of Maximum Heart Rate

**AGE** 15 20 25 30 35 40 45 50 55 60 65 70 75 80

Warm Up · Beginner · Intermediate · Advanced · Sprint Pace

AEROBIC · ANAEROBIC

# MUSCLE GROUPS

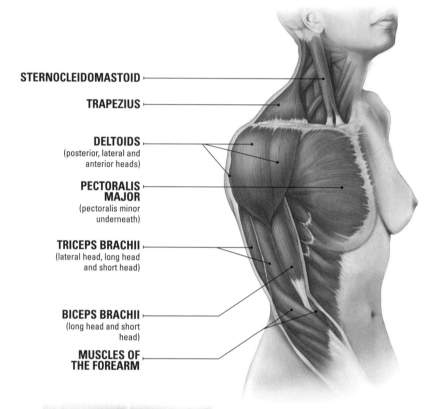

STERNOCLEIDOMASTOID

TRAPEZIUS

**DELTOIDS**
(posterior, lateral and anterior heads)

**PECTORALIS MAJOR**
(pectoralis minor underneath)

**TRICEPS BRACHII**
(lateral head, long head and short head)

**BICEPS BRACHII**
(long head and short head)

**MUSCLES OF THE FOREARM**

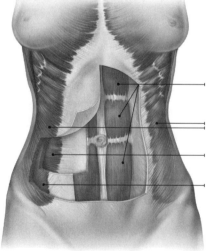

RECTUS ABDOMINIS

EXTERNAL OBLIQUES

TRANSVERSUS ABDOMINIS

INTERNAL OBLIQUES

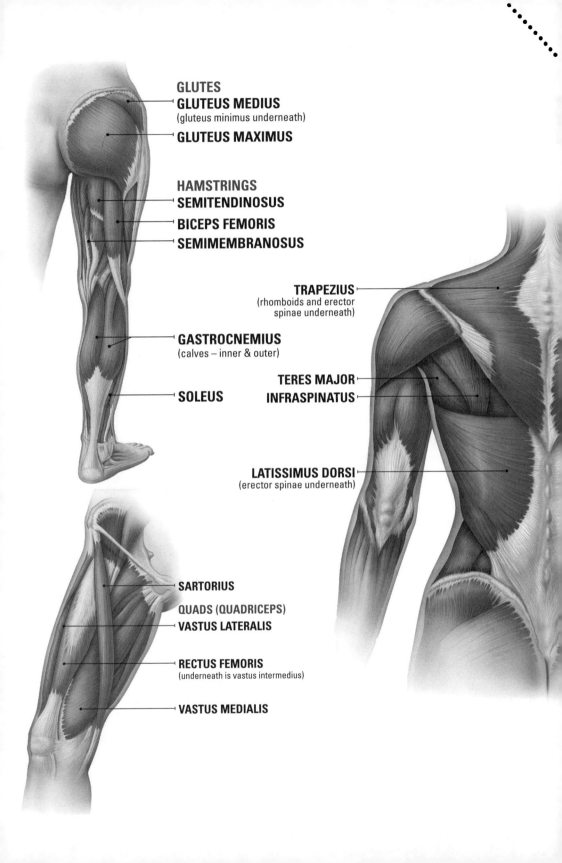

GLUTES
**GLUTEUS MEDIUS**
(gluteus minimus underneath)

**GLUTEUS MAXIMUS**

HAMSTRINGS
**SEMITENDINOSUS**

**BICEPS FEMORIS**

**SEMIMEMBRANOSUS**

**TRAPEZIUS**
(rhomboids and erector
spinae underneath)

**GASTROCNEMIUS**
(calves – inner & outer)

**TERES MAJOR**
**INFRASPINATUS**

**SOLEUS**

**LATISSIMUS DORSI**
(erector spinae underneath)

**SARTORIUS**

QUADS (QUADRICEPS)
**VASTUS LATERALIS**

**RECTUS FEMORIS**
(underneath is vastus intermedius)

**VASTUS MEDIALIS**

# PERSONAL DATA

|  | DATE | DATE | DATE |
|---|---|---|---|
| **WEIGHT** | | | |
| **BODY-FAT PERCENTAGE** | | | |

## MEASUREMENTS

|  | | | |
|---|---|---|---|
| **CHEST** | | | |
| **WAIST** | | | |
| **HIPS** | | | |
| **THIGH** | | | |
| **RIGHT ARM** - relaxed: | | | |
| - flexed: | | | |
| **LEFT ARM** - relaxed: | | | |
| - flexed: | | | |
| **RIGHT CALF** | | | |
| **LEFT CALF** | | | |
| **NECK** | | | |
| **FOREARM** | | | |

|  | DATE | DATE | DATE |
|---|---|---|---|
| **WEIGHT** | | | |
| **BODY-FAT PERCENTAGE** | | | |

## MEASUREMENTS

|  |  |  |  |
|---|---|---|---|
| **CHEST** | | | |
| **WAIST** | | | |
| **HIPS** | | | |
| **THIGH** | | | |
| **RIGHT ARM** <br> - relaxed: | | | |
| - flexed: | | | |
| **LEFT ARM** <br> - relaxed: | | | |
| - flexed: | | | |
| **RIGHT CALF** | | | |
| **LEFT CALF** | | | |
| **NECK** | | | |
| **FOREARM** | | | |

# GOALS

Setting goals is the key to success. Each goal is a stepping stone toward your ideal self. Give yourself reasonable goals to work toward. Rather than trying to lose 20 lbs. in one week, strive for 2 lbs. You can try for 20 lbs. over time.

Breaking your long-term goal into attainable short-term goals keeps you aware of your progress, and you are constantly rewarding yourself by completing one step toward a better you!

## WEEKLY GOALS

Making positive changes each week will add up. You'll start seeing results in no time!
By this time next week...

## MONTHLY GOALS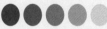

Some of your goals will take a little longer. Choose a few monthly goals and stick to the changes you've already made.
By this time next month...

## LONG-TERM GOALS

Studies have shown that people who write down their long-term goals are more successful in many aspects of life than those who do not. Do it now!
By this time next year...

# GOALS

Setting goals is the key to success. Each goal is a stepping stone toward your ideal self. Give yourself reasonable goals to work toward. Rather than trying to lose 20 lbs. in one week, strive for 2 lbs. You can try for 20 lbs. over time.

Breaking your long-term goal into attainable short-term goals keeps you aware of your progress, and you are constantly rewarding yourself by completing one step toward a better you!

## WEEKLY GOALS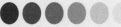

Making positive changes each week will add up. You'll start seeing results in no time!
By this time next week...

## MONTHLY GOALS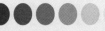

Some of your goals will take a little longer. Choose a few monthly goals and stick to the changes you've already made.
By this time next month...

## LONG-TERM GOALS

Studies have shown that people who write down their long-term goals are more successful in many aspects of life than those who do not. Do it now!
By this time next year...

# GOALS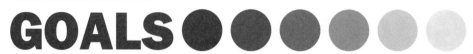

Setting goals is the key to success. Each goal is a stepping stone toward your ideal self. Give yourself reasonable goals to work toward. Rather than trying to lose 20 lbs. in one week, strive for 2 lbs. You can try for 20 lbs. over time.

Breaking your long-term goal into attainable short-term goals keeps you aware of your progress, and you are constantly rewarding yourself by completing one step toward a better you!

## WEEKLY GOALS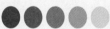

Making positive changes each week will add up. You'll start seeing results in no time!
By this time next week...

## MONTHLY GOALS

Some of your goals will take a little longer. Choose a few monthly goals and stick to the changes you've already made.
By this time next month...

## LONG-TERM GOALS

Studies have shown that people who write down their long-term goals are more successful in many aspects of life than those who do not. Do it now!
By this time next year...

# GOALS

Setting goals is the key to success. Each goal is a stepping stone toward your ideal self. Give yourself reasonable goals to work toward. Rather than trying to lose 20 lbs. in one week, strive for 2 lbs. You can try for 20 lbs. over time.

Breaking your long-term goal into attainable short-term goals keeps you aware of your progress, and you are constantly rewarding yourself by completing one step toward a better you!

## WEEKLY GOALS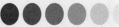

Making positive changes each week will add up. You'll start seeing results in no time!
By this time next week...

## MONTHLY GOALS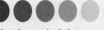

Some of your goals will take a little longer. Choose a few monthly goals and stick to the changes you've already made.
By this time next month...

## LONG-TERM GOALS ●●●●●●

Studies have shown that people who write down their long-term goals are more successful in many aspects of life than those who do not. Do it now!
By this time next year...

# GOALS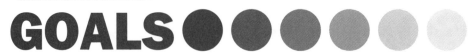

Setting goals is the key to success. Each goal is a stepping stone toward your ideal self. Give yourself reasonable goals to work toward. Rather than trying to lose 20 lbs. in one week, strive for 2 lbs. You can try for 20 lbs. over time.

Breaking your long-term goal into attainable short-term goals keeps you aware of your progress, and you are constantly rewarding yourself by completing one step toward a better you!

## WEEKLY GOALS

Making positive changes each week will add up. You'll start seeing results in no time!
By this time next week...

## MONTHLY GOALS

Some of your goals will take a little longer. Choose a few monthly goals and stick to the changes you've already made.
By this time next month...

## LONG-TERM GOALS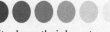

Studies have shown that people who write down their long-term goals are more successful in many aspects of life than those who do not. Do it now!
By this time next year...

# GOALS

Setting goals is the key to success. Each goal is a stepping stone toward your ideal self. Give yourself reasonable goals to work toward. Rather than trying to lose 20 lbs. in one week, strive for 2 lbs. You can try for 20 lbs. over time.

Breaking your long-term goal into attainable short-term goals keeps you aware of your progress, and you are constantly rewarding yourself by completing one step toward a better you!

## WEEKLY GOALS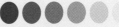

Making positive changes each week will add up. You'll start seeing results in no time!
By this time next week...

## MONTHLY GOALS

Some of your goals will take a little longer. Choose a few monthly goals and stick to the changes you've already made.
By this time next month...

## LONG-TERM GOALS

Studies have shown that people who write down their long-term goals are more successful in many aspects of life than those who do not. Do it now!
By this time next year...

# YOUR TRAINING
# JOURNAL

DATE [            ]

| EXERCISE | | SET 1 | SET 2 | SET 3 | SET 4 | SET 5 | SET 6 |
|---|---|---|---|---|---|---|---|
| | WEIGHT | | | | | | |
| | REPS | | | | | | |
| | WEIGHT | | | | | | |
| | REPS | | | | | | |
| | WEIGHT | | | | | | |
| | REPS | | | | | | |
| | WEIGHT | | | | | | |
| | REPS | | | | | | |
| | WEIGHT | | | | | | |
| | REPS | | | | | | |
| | WEIGHT | | | | | | |
| | REPS | | | | | | |
| | WEIGHT | | | | | | |
| | REPS | | | | | | |
| | WEIGHT | | | | | | |
| | REPS | | | | | | |
| | WEIGHT | | | | | | |
| | REPS | | | | | | |
| | WEIGHT | | | | | | |
| | REPS | | | | | | |
| | WEIGHT | | | | | | |
| | REPS | | | | | | |

**CARDIO ACTIVITY:**

**NOTES:**

## TIP

Abs are used to stabilize the legs and torso during all exercises. Train abs at the end so as not to fatigue them early.

# YOUR TRAINING
# JOURNAL

**DATE**

| EXERCISE | | SET 1 | SET 2 | SET 3 | SET 4 | SET 5 | SET 6 |
|---|---|---|---|---|---|---|---|
| | WEIGHT | | | | | | |
| | REPS | | | | | | |
| | WEIGHT | | | | | | |
| | REPS | | | | | | |
| | WEIGHT | | | | | | |
| | REPS | | | | | | |
| | WEIGHT | | | | | | |
| | REPS | | | | | | |
| | WEIGHT | | | | | | |
| | REPS | | | | | | |
| | WEIGHT | | | | | | |
| | REPS | | | | | | |
| | WEIGHT | | | | | | |
| | REPS | | | | | | |
| | WEIGHT | | | | | | |
| | REPS | | | | | | |
| | WEIGHT | | | | | | |
| | REPS | | | | | | |
| | WEIGHT | | | | | | |
| | REPS | | | | | | |
| | WEIGHT | | | | | | |
| | REPS | | | | | | |

**CARDIO ACTIVITY:**

**NOTES:**

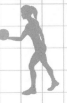

## TIP
Muscle loves to eat fat! The more muscle you have
the leaner you will become.

# YOUR TRAINING JOURNAL

DATE

| EXERCISE | | SET 1 | SET 2 | SET 3 | SET 4 | SET 5 | SET 6 |
|---|---|---|---|---|---|---|---|
| | WEIGHT | | | | | | |
| | REPS | | | | | | |
| | WEIGHT | | | | | | |
| | REPS | | | | | | |
| | WEIGHT | | | | | | |
| | REPS | | | | | | |
| | WEIGHT | | | | | | |
| | REPS | | | | | | |
| | WEIGHT | | | | | | |
| | REPS | | | | | | |
| | WEIGHT | | | | | | |
| | REPS | | | | | | |
| | WEIGHT | | | | | | |
| | REPS | | | | | | |
| | WEIGHT | | | | | | |
| | REPS | | | | | | |
| | WEIGHT | | | | | | |
| | REPS | | | | | | |
| | WEIGHT | | | | | | |
| | REPS | | | | | | |
| | WEIGHT | | | | | | |
| | REPS | | | | | | |

**CARDIO ACTIVITY:**

**NOTES:**

## TIP

Bison is an excellent lean protein source with a better nutritional profile than beef. Tastes delicious too!

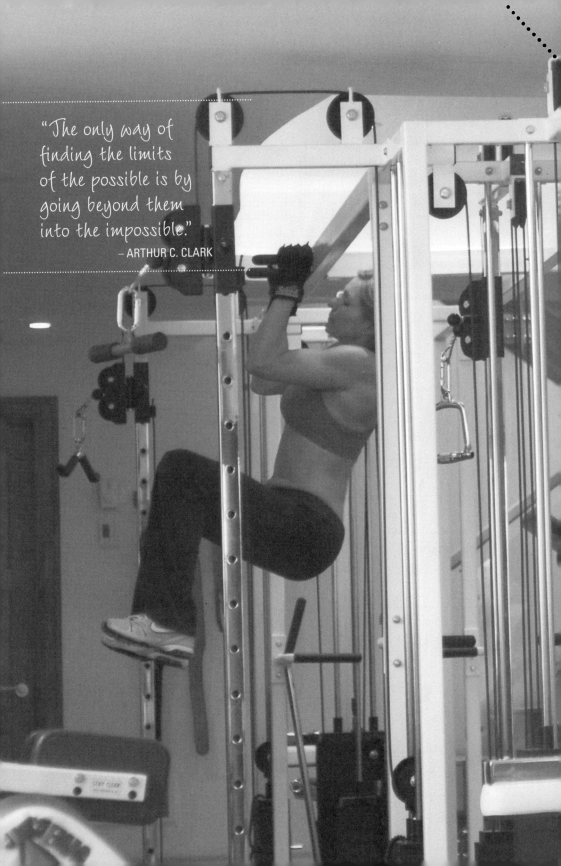

"The only way of finding the limits of the possible is by going beyond them into the impossible."
— ARTHUR C. CLARK

# YOUR TRAINING
# JOURNAL

DATE

| EXERCISE | | SET 1 | SET 2 | SET 3 | SET 4 | SET 5 | SET 6 |
|---|---|---|---|---|---|---|---|
| | WEIGHT | | | | | | |
| | REPS | | | | | | |
| | WEIGHT | | | | | | |
| | REPS | | | | | | |
| | WEIGHT | | | | | | |
| | REPS | | | | | | |
| | WEIGHT | | | | | | |
| | REPS | | | | | | |
| | WEIGHT | | | | | | |
| | REPS | | | | | | |
| | WEIGHT | | | | | | |
| | REPS | | | | | | |
| | WEIGHT | | | | | | |
| | REPS | | | | | | |
| | WEIGHT | | | | | | |
| | REPS | | | | | | |
| | WEIGHT | | | | | | |
| | REPS | | | | | | |
| | WEIGHT | | | | | | |
| | REPS | | | | | | |
| | WEIGHT | | | | | | |
| | REPS | | | | | | |

**CARDIO ACTIVITY:**

**NOTES:**

## TIP
Clean out your cupboards. Make sure to get rid of all your trouble foods. They are sticking points.

# YOUR TRAINING JOURNAL

**DATE**

| EXERCISE | | SET 1 | SET 2 | SET 3 | SET 4 | SET 5 | SET 6 |
|---|---|---|---|---|---|---|---|
| | WEIGHT | | | | | | |
| | REPS | | | | | | |
| | WEIGHT | | | | | | |
| | REPS | | | | | | |
| | WEIGHT | | | | | | |
| | REPS | | | | | | |
| | WEIGHT | | | | | | |
| | REPS | | | | | | |
| | WEIGHT | | | | | | |
| | REPS | | | | | | |
| | WEIGHT | | | | | | |
| | REPS | | | | | | |
| | WEIGHT | | | | | | |
| | REPS | | | | | | |
| | WEIGHT | | | | | | |
| | REPS | | | | | | |
| | WEIGHT | | | | | | |
| | REPS | | | | | | |
| | WEIGHT | | | | | | |
| | REPS | | | | | | |
| | WEIGHT | | | | | | |
| | REPS | | | | | | |

**CARDIO ACTIVITY:**

**NOTES:**

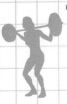

**TIP**
Drink green tea for antioxidants, flavonoids and natural fat-burning agents.

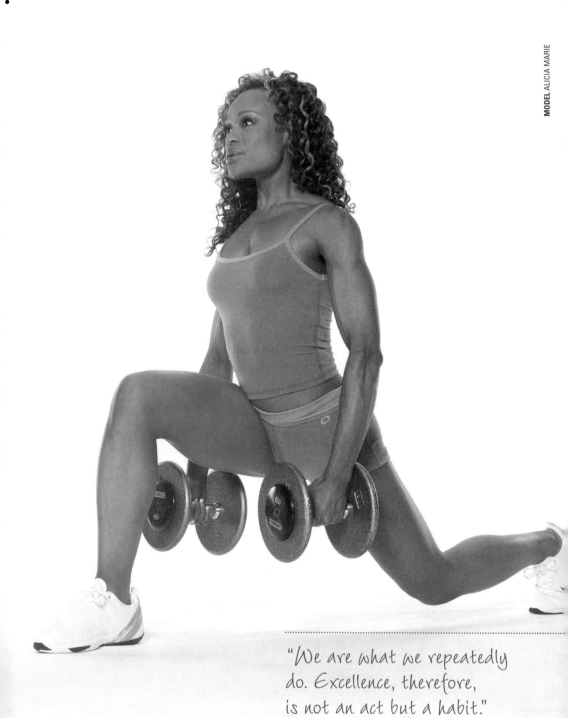

"We are what we repeatedly
do. Excellence, therefore,
is not an act but a habit."

– ARISTOTLE

# YOUR TRAINING JOURNAL

**DATE**

| EXERCISE | | SET 1 | SET 2 | SET 3 | SET 4 | SET 5 | SET 6 |
|---|---|---|---|---|---|---|---|
| | WEIGHT | | | | | | |
| | REPS | | | | | | |
| | WEIGHT | | | | | | |
| | REPS | | | | | | |
| | WEIGHT | | | | | | |
| | REPS | | | | | | |
| | WEIGHT | | | | | | |
| | REPS | | | | | | |
| | WEIGHT | | | | | | |
| | REPS | | | | | | |
| | WEIGHT | | | | | | |
| | REPS | | | | | | |
| | WEIGHT | | | | | | |
| | REPS | | | | | | |
| | WEIGHT | | | | | | |
| | REPS | | | | | | |
| | WEIGHT | | | | | | |
| | REPS | | | | | | |
| | WEIGHT | | | | | | |
| | REPS | | | | | | |
| | WEIGHT | | | | | | |
| | REPS | | | | | | |

**CARDIO ACTIVITY:**

**NOTES:**

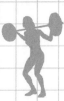

## TIP

Add one tablespoon of lightly ground flaxseed to your morning cereal or smoothie. Flaxseed is excellent for EFAs (healthy fats), lignins, and fiber, which helps move lazy bowels.

# YOUR TRAINING
# JOURNAL

**DATE**

| EXERCISE | | SET 1 | SET 2 | SET 3 | SET 4 | SET 5 | SET 6 |
|---|---|---|---|---|---|---|---|
| | WEIGHT | | | | | | |
| | REPS | | | | | | |
| | WEIGHT | | | | | | |
| | REPS | | | | | | |
| | WEIGHT | | | | | | |
| | REPS | | | | | | |
| | WEIGHT | | | | | | |
| | REPS | | | | | | |
| | WEIGHT | | | | | | |
| | REPS | | | | | | |
| | WEIGHT | | | | | | |
| | REPS | | | | | | |
| | WEIGHT | | | | | | |
| | REPS | | | | | | |
| | WEIGHT | | | | | | |
| | REPS | | | | | | |
| | WEIGHT | | | | | | |
| | REPS | | | | | | |
| | WEIGHT | | | | | | |
| | REPS | | | | | | |
| | WEIGHT | | | | | | |
| | REPS | | | | | | |

**CARDIO ACTIVITY:**

**NOTES:**

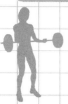

## TIP

Training is your time. Don't answer the phone or allow distractions. This is all about you!

# YOUR TRAINING JOURNAL

DATE

| EXERCISE | | SET 1 | SET 2 | SET 3 | SET 4 | SET 5 | SET 6 |
|----------|---|-------|-------|-------|-------|-------|-------|
| | WEIGHT | | | | | | |
| | REPS | | | | | | |
| | WEIGHT | | | | | | |
| | REPS | | | | | | |
| | WEIGHT | | | | | | |
| | REPS | | | | | | |
| | WEIGHT | | | | | | |
| | REPS | | | | | | |
| | WEIGHT | | | | | | |
| | REPS | | | | | | |
| | WEIGHT | | | | | | |
| | REPS | | | | | | |
| | WEIGHT | | | | | | |
| | REPS | | | | | | |
| | WEIGHT | | | | | | |
| | REPS | | | | | | |
| | WEIGHT | | | | | | |
| | REPS | | | | | | |
| | WEIGHT | | | | | | |
| | REPS | | | | | | |
| | WEIGHT | | | | | | |
| | REPS | | | | | | |

**CARDIO ACTIVITY:**

**NOTES:**

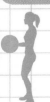

## TIP

Jo keep your heart rate high while weight training, reduce rest time between sets.

# YOUR TRAINING
# JOURNAL

**DATE**

| EXERCISE | | SET 1 | SET 2 | SET 3 | SET 4 | SET 5 | SET 6 |
|---|---|---|---|---|---|---|---|
| | WEIGHT | | | | | | |
| | REPS | | | | | | |
| | WEIGHT | | | | | | |
| | REPS | | | | | | |
| | WEIGHT | | | | | | |
| | REPS | | | | | | |
| | WEIGHT | | | | | | |
| | REPS | | | | | | |
| | WEIGHT | | | | | | |
| | REPS | | | | | | |
| | WEIGHT | | | | | | |
| | REPS | | | | | | |
| | WEIGHT | | | | | | |
| | REPS | | | | | | |
| | WEIGHT | | | | | | |
| | REPS | | | | | | |
| | WEIGHT | | | | | | |
| | REPS | | | | | | |
| | WEIGHT | | | | | | |
| | REPS | | | | | | |
| | WEIGHT | | | | | | |
| | REPS | | | | | | |

**CARDIO ACTIVITY:**

**NOTES:**

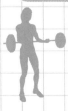

## TIP
Accelerate fat loss by skipping rope between your sets for your entire workout.

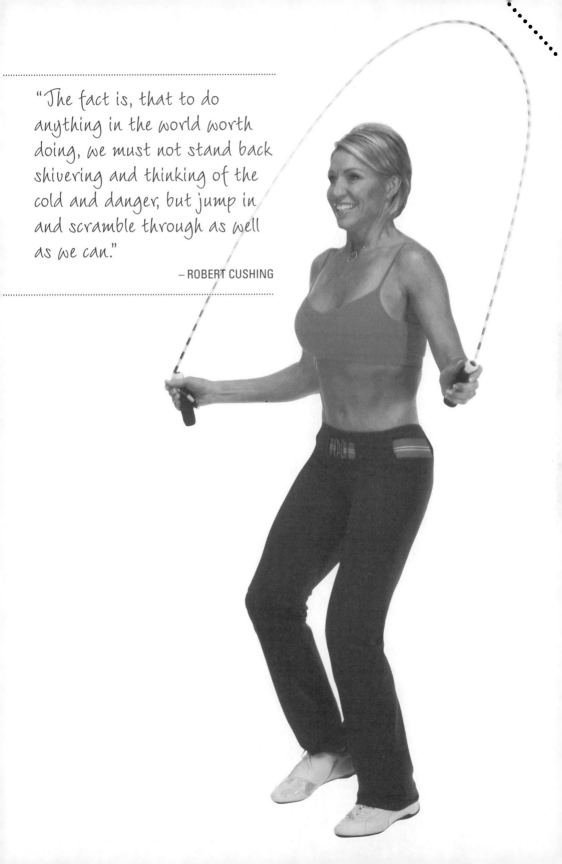

"The fact is, that to do anything in the world worth doing, we must not stand back shivering and thinking of the cold and danger, but jump in and scramble through as well as we can."

– ROBERT CUSHING

# YOUR TRAINING
# JOURNAL

DATE

| EXERCISE | | SET 1 | SET 2 | SET 3 | SET 4 | SET 5 | SET 6 |
|---|---|---|---|---|---|---|---|
| | WEIGHT | | | | | | |
| | REPS | | | | | | |
| | WEIGHT | | | | | | |
| | REPS | | | | | | |
| | WEIGHT | | | | | | |
| | REPS | | | | | | |
| | WEIGHT | | | | | | |
| | REPS | | | | | | |
| | WEIGHT | | | | | | |
| | REPS | | | | | | |
| | WEIGHT | | | | | | |
| | REPS | | | | | | |
| | WEIGHT | | | | | | |
| | REPS | | | | | | |
| | WEIGHT | | | | | | |
| | REPS | | | | | | |
| | WEIGHT | | | | | | |
| | REPS | | | | | | |
| | WEIGHT | | | | | | |
| | REPS | | | | | | |
| | WEIGHT | | | | | | |
| | REPS | | | | | | |

**CARDIO ACTIVITY:**

**NOTES:**

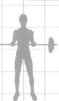

## TIP
Stress is a killer and it generates belly fat. Blast it away by making training a priority three to five times per week.

# YOUR TRAINING JOURNAL

**DATE**

| EXERCISE | | SET 1 | SET 2 | SET 3 | SET 4 | SET 5 | SET 6 |
|---|---|---|---|---|---|---|---|
| | WEIGHT | | | | | | |
| | REPS | | | | | | |
| | WEIGHT | | | | | | |
| | REPS | | | | | | |
| | WEIGHT | | | | | | |
| | REPS | | | | | | |
| | WEIGHT | | | | | | |
| | REPS | | | | | | |
| | WEIGHT | | | | | | |
| | REPS | | | | | | |
| | WEIGHT | | | | | | |
| | REPS | | | | | | |
| | WEIGHT | | | | | | |
| | REPS | | | | | | |
| | WEIGHT | | | | | | |
| | REPS | | | | | | |
| | WEIGHT | | | | | | |
| | REPS | | | | | | |
| | WEIGHT | | | | | | |
| | REPS | | | | | | |
| | WEIGHT | | | | | | |
| | REPS | | | | | | |

**CARDIO ACTIVITY:**

**NOTES:**

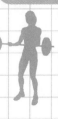

## TIP
Water is absolutely essential during regular activities but especially during training. Drink two to three liters per day.

# YOUR TRAINING JOURNAL

DATE

| EXERCISE | | SET 1 | SET 2 | SET 3 | SET 4 | SET 5 | SET 6 |
|---|---|---|---|---|---|---|---|
| | WEIGHT | | | | | | |
| | REPS | | | | | | |
| | WEIGHT | | | | | | |
| | REPS | | | | | | |
| | WEIGHT | | | | | | |
| | REPS | | | | | | |
| | WEIGHT | | | | | | |
| | REPS | | | | | | |
| | WEIGHT | | | | | | |
| | REPS | | | | | | |
| | WEIGHT | | | | | | |
| | REPS | | | | | | |
| | WEIGHT | | | | | | |
| | REPS | | | | | | |
| | WEIGHT | | | | | | |
| | REPS | | | | | | |
| | WEIGHT | | | | | | |
| | REPS | | | | | | |
| | WEIGHT | | | | | | |
| | REPS | | | | | | |
| | WEIGHT | | | | | | |
| | REPS | | | | | | |

**CARDIO ACTIVITY:**

**NOTES:**

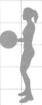

## TIP

Don't make excuses to skip your workout. Training is a privilege, not a punishment.

# YOUR TRAINING
# JOURNAL

**DATE**

| EXERCISE | | SET 1 | SET 2 | SET 3 | SET 4 | SET 5 | SET 6 |
|---|---|---|---|---|---|---|---|
| | WEIGHT | | | | | | |
| | REPS | | | | | | |
| | WEIGHT | | | | | | |
| | REPS | | | | | | |
| | WEIGHT | | | | | | |
| | REPS | | | | | | |
| | WEIGHT | | | | | | |
| | REPS | | | | | | |
| | WEIGHT | | | | | | |
| | REPS | | | | | | |
| | WEIGHT | | | | | | |
| | REPS | | | | | | |
| | WEIGHT | | | | | | |
| | REPS | | | | | | |
| | WEIGHT | | | | | | |
| | REPS | | | | | | |
| | WEIGHT | | | | | | |
| | REPS | | | | | | |
| | WEIGHT | | | | | | |
| | REPS | | | | | | |
| | WEIGHT | | | | | | |
| | REPS | | | | | | |

**CARDIO ACTIVITY:**

**NOTES:**

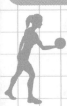

## TIP
Skipping a meal is worse than skipping a workout. Eat six meals a day, every day!

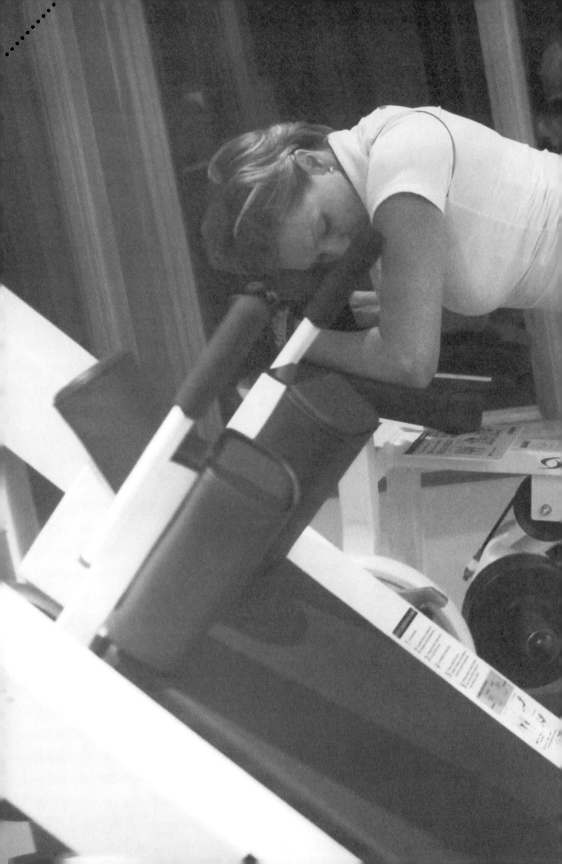

"Nothing will ever be attempted if all possible objections must first be overcome."

– SAMUEL JOHNSON

# YOUR TRAINING
# JOURNAL

DATE

| EXERCISE | | SET 1 | SET 2 | SET 3 | SET 4 | SET 5 | SET 6 |
|---|---|---|---|---|---|---|---|
| | WEIGHT | | | | | | |
| | REPS | | | | | | |
| | WEIGHT | | | | | | |
| | REPS | | | | | | |
| | WEIGHT | | | | | | |
| | REPS | | | | | | |
| | WEIGHT | | | | | | |
| | REPS | | | | | | |
| | WEIGHT | | | | | | |
| | REPS | | | | | | |
| | WEIGHT | | | | | | |
| | REPS | | | | | | |
| | WEIGHT | | | | | | |
| | REPS | | | | | | |
| | WEIGHT | | | | | | |
| | REPS | | | | | | |
| | WEIGHT | | | | | | |
| | REPS | | | | | | |
| | WEIGHT | | | | | | |
| | REPS | | | | | | |
| | WEIGHT | | | | | | |
| | REPS | | | | | | |

**CARDIO ACTIVITY:**

**NOTES:**

## TIP

Remove processed food from your diet. If you can't recognize ingredients on the label, don't eat it.

# YOUR TRAINING
# JOURNAL

DATE 

| EXERCISE | | SET 1 | SET 2 | SET 3 | SET 4 | SET 5 | SET 6 |
|---|---|---|---|---|---|---|---|
| | WEIGHT | | | | | | |
| | REPS | | | | | | |
| | WEIGHT | | | | | | |
| | REPS | | | | | | |
| | WEIGHT | | | | | | |
| | REPS | | | | | | |
| | WEIGHT | | | | | | |
| | REPS | | | | | | |
| | WEIGHT | | | | | | |
| | REPS | | | | | | |
| | WEIGHT | | | | | | |
| | REPS | | | | | | |
| | WEIGHT | | | | | | |
| | REPS | | | | | | |
| | WEIGHT | | | | | | |
| | REPS | | | | | | |
| | WEIGHT | | | | | | |
| | REPS | | | | | | |
| | WEIGHT | | | | | | |
| | REPS | | | | | | |
| | WEIGHT | | | | | | |
| | REPS | | | | | | |

**CARDIO ACTIVITY:**

**NOTES:**

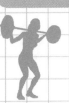

**TIP**
Eat brown rice rather than white. It has a higher nutritional profile and tastes better too.

# YOUR TRAINING
# JOURNAL

DATE

| EXERCISE | | SET 1 | SET 2 | SET 3 | SET 4 | SET 5 | SET 6 |
|---|---|---|---|---|---|---|---|
| | WEIGHT | | | | | | |
| | REPS | | | | | | |
| | WEIGHT | | | | | | |
| | REPS | | | | | | |
| | WEIGHT | | | | | | |
| | REPS | | | | | | |
| | WEIGHT | | | | | | |
| | REPS | | | | | | |
| | WEIGHT | | | | | | |
| | REPS | | | | | | |
| | WEIGHT | | | | | | |
| | REPS | | | | | | |
| | WEIGHT | | | | | | |
| | REPS | | | | | | |
| | WEIGHT | | | | | | |
| | REPS | | | | | | |
| | WEIGHT | | | | | | |
| | REPS | | | | | | |
| | WEIGHT | | | | | | |
| | REPS | | | | | | |
| | WEIGHT | | | | | | |
| | REPS | | | | | | |

**CARDIO ACTIVITY:**

**NOTES:**

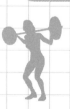

## TIP

Eat foods rich in CLA — conjugated linoleic acid. CLA is a natural fat-burning chemical in the body. Try chlorella, spirulina and blue-green algae.

# YOUR TRAINING JOURNAL

DATE

| EXERCISE | | SET 1 | SET 2 | SET 3 | SET 4 | SET 5 | SET 6 |
|---|---|---|---|---|---|---|---|
| | WEIGHT | | | | | | |
| | REPS | | | | | | |
| | WEIGHT | | | | | | |
| | REPS | | | | | | |
| | WEIGHT | | | | | | |
| | REPS | | | | | | |
| | WEIGHT | | | | | | |
| | REPS | | | | | | |
| | WEIGHT | | | | | | |
| | REPS | | | | | | |
| | WEIGHT | | | | | | |
| | REPS | | | | | | |
| | WEIGHT | | | | | | |
| | REPS | | | | | | |
| | WEIGHT | | | | | | |
| | REPS | | | | | | |
| | WEIGHT | | | | | | |
| | REPS | | | | | | |
| | WEIGHT | | | | | | |
| | REPS | | | | | | |
| | WEIGHT | | | | | | |
| | REPS | | | | | | |

**CARDIO ACTIVITY:**

**NOTES:**

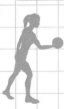

## TIP
Introduce a variety of healthy oils (fats) into your diet. My favorites are pumpkinseed, olive, avocado, rice bran and tomato-seed oils.

# YOUR TRAINING JOURNAL

DATE

| EXERCISE | | SET 1 | SET 2 | SET 3 | SET 4 | SET 5 | SET 6 |
|---|---|---|---|---|---|---|---|
| | WEIGHT | | | | | | |
| | REPS | | | | | | |
| | WEIGHT | | | | | | |
| | REPS | | | | | | |
| | WEIGHT | | | | | | |
| | REPS | | | | | | |
| | WEIGHT | | | | | | |
| | REPS | | | | | | |
| | WEIGHT | | | | | | |
| | REPS | | | | | | |
| | WEIGHT | | | | | | |
| | REPS | | | | | | |
| | WEIGHT | | | | | | |
| | REPS | | | | | | |
| | WEIGHT | | | | | | |
| | REPS | | | | | | |
| | WEIGHT | | | | | | |
| | REPS | | | | | | |
| | WEIGHT | | | | | | |
| | REPS | | | | | | |
| | WEIGHT | | | | | | |
| | REPS | | | | | | |

**CARDIO ACTIVITY:**

**NOTES:**

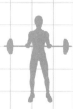

## TIP
Drink your coffee black. Eliminating sugar and cream from a "regular" or loaded coffee will cut fat from your diet right away.

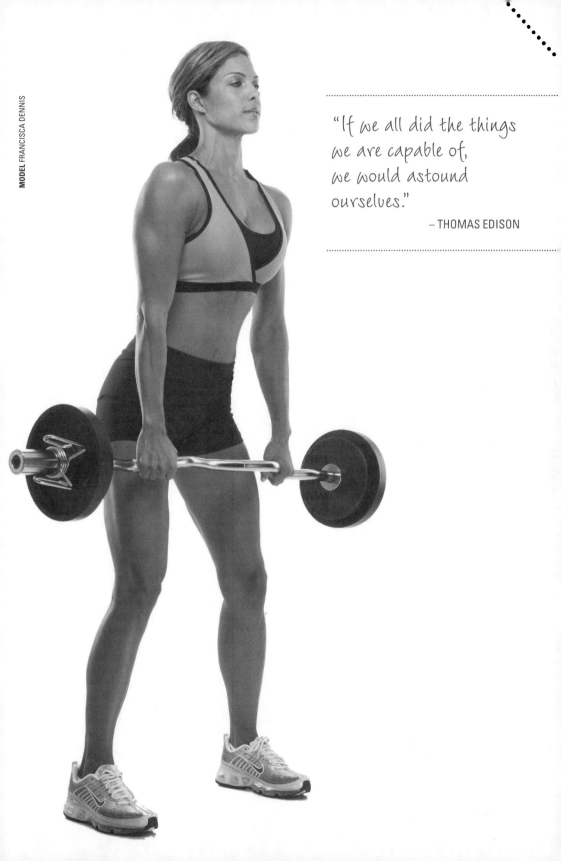

"If we all did the things
we are capable of,
we would astound
ourselves."

– THOMAS EDISON

# YOUR TRAINING
# JOURNAL

DATE

| EXERCISE | | SET 1 | SET 2 | SET 3 | SET 4 | SET 5 | SET 6 |
|---|---|---|---|---|---|---|---|
| | WEIGHT | | | | | | |
| | REPS | | | | | | |
| | WEIGHT | | | | | | |
| | REPS | | | | | | |
| | WEIGHT | | | | | | |
| | REPS | | | | | | |
| | WEIGHT | | | | | | |
| | REPS | | | | | | |
| | WEIGHT | | | | | | |
| | REPS | | | | | | |
| | WEIGHT | | | | | | |
| | REPS | | | | | | |
| | WEIGHT | | | | | | |
| | REPS | | | | | | |
| | WEIGHT | | | | | | |
| | REPS | | | | | | |
| | WEIGHT | | | | | | |
| | REPS | | | | | | |
| | WEIGHT | | | | | | |
| | REPS | | | | | | |
| | WEIGHT | | | | | | |
| | REPS | | | | | | |

**CARDIO ACTIVITY:**

**NOTES:**

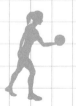

## TIP

Sanitize your hands after every workout. Use an alcohol-based sanitizer and avoid the deadly MRSA bug. I carry a purse-sized sanitizer with me all the time.

# YOUR TRAINING
# JOURNAL

**DATE**

| EXERCISE | | SET 1 | SET 2 | SET 3 | SET 4 | SET 5 | SET 6 |
|---|---|---|---|---|---|---|---|
| | WEIGHT | | | | | | |
| | REPS | | | | | | |
| | WEIGHT | | | | | | |
| | REPS | | | | | | |
| | WEIGHT | | | | | | |
| | REPS | | | | | | |
| | WEIGHT | | | | | | |
| | REPS | | | | | | |
| | WEIGHT | | | | | | |
| | REPS | | | | | | |
| | WEIGHT | | | | | | |
| | REPS | | | | | | |
| | WEIGHT | | | | | | |
| | REPS | | | | | | |
| | WEIGHT | | | | | | |
| | REPS | | | | | | |
| | WEIGHT | | | | | | |
| | REPS | | | | | | |
| | WEIGHT | | | | | | |
| | REPS | | | | | | |
| | WEIGHT | | | | | | |
| | REPS | | | | | | |

**CARDIO ACTIVITY:**

**NOTES:**

## TIP
*When doing any exercise, concentrate on the muscle group you are working and contract your abs, too!*

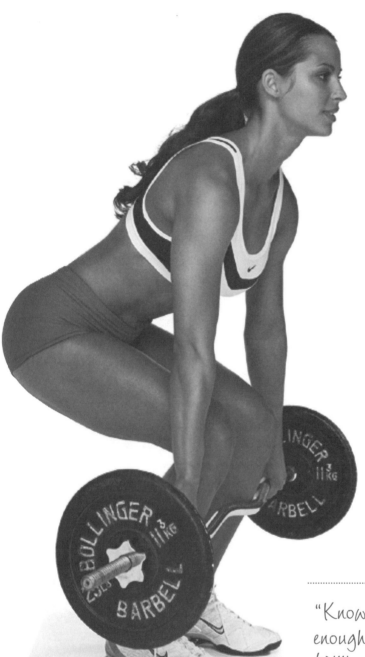

"Knowing is not
enough; we must apply.
Willing is not enough;
we must do."
– JOHANN WOLFGANG VON GOETHE

# YOUR TRAINING
# JOURNAL

DATE

| EXERCISE | | SET 1 | SET 2 | SET 3 | SET 4 | SET 5 | SET 6 |
|---|---|---|---|---|---|---|---|
| | WEIGHT | | | | | | |
| | REPS | | | | | | |
| | WEIGHT | | | | | | |
| | REPS | | | | | | |
| | WEIGHT | | | | | | |
| | REPS | | | | | | |
| | WEIGHT | | | | | | |
| | REPS | | | | | | |
| | WEIGHT | | | | | | |
| | REPS | | | | | | |
| | WEIGHT | | | | | | |
| | REPS | | | | | | |
| | WEIGHT | | | | | | |
| | REPS | | | | | | |
| | WEIGHT | | | | | | |
| | REPS | | | | | | |
| | WEIGHT | | | | | | |
| | REPS | | | | | | |
| | WEIGHT | | | | | | |
| | REPS | | | | | | |
| | WEIGHT | | | | | | |
| | REPS | | | | | | |

**CARDIO ACTIVITY:**

**NOTES:**

## TIP

Mix up your cardio. Don't run every day. Alternate cardio activity by mixing it up every few days with activities such as running bleachers, rope jumping, swimming, cardio, kick boxing or any other physical activity.

# YOUR TRAINING
# JOURNAL

DATE

| EXERCISE | | SET 1 | SET 2 | SET 3 | SET 4 | SET 5 | SET 6 |
|---|---|---|---|---|---|---|---|
| | WEIGHT | | | | | | |
| | REPS | | | | | | |
| | WEIGHT | | | | | | |
| | REPS | | | | | | |
| | WEIGHT | | | | | | |
| | REPS | | | | | | |
| | WEIGHT | | | | | | |
| | REPS | | | | | | |
| | WEIGHT | | | | | | |
| | REPS | | | | | | |
| | WEIGHT | | | | | | |
| | REPS | | | | | | |
| | WEIGHT | | | | | | |
| | REPS | | | | | | |
| | WEIGHT | | | | | | |
| | REPS | | | | | | |
| | WEIGHT | | | | | | |
| | REPS | | | | | | |
| | WEIGHT | | | | | | |
| | REPS | | | | | | |
| | WEIGHT | | | | | | |
| | REPS | | | | | | |

**CARDIO ACTIVITY:**

**NOTES:**

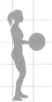

## TIP
Use a small towel on the benches and equipment you are using at the gym. This keeps the bench dry and is proper gym etiquette to accommodate the next person using the equipment.

# YOUR TRAINING JOURNAL

DATE

| EXERCISE | | SET 1 | SET 2 | SET 3 | SET 4 | SET 5 | SET 6 |
|---|---|---|---|---|---|---|---|
| | WEIGHT | | | | | | |
| | REPS | | | | | | |
| | WEIGHT | | | | | | |
| | REPS | | | | | | |
| | WEIGHT | | | | | | |
| | REPS | | | | | | |
| | WEIGHT | | | | | | |
| | REPS | | | | | | |
| | WEIGHT | | | | | | |
| | REPS | | | | | | |
| | WEIGHT | | | | | | |
| | REPS | | | | | | |
| | WEIGHT | | | | | | |
| | REPS | | | | | | |
| | WEIGHT | | | | | | |
| | REPS | | | | | | |
| | WEIGHT | | | | | | |
| | REPS | | | | | | |
| | WEIGHT | | | | | | |
| | REPS | | | | | | |
| | WEIGHT | | | | | | |
| | REPS | | | | | | |

**CARDIO ACTIVITY:**

**NOTES:**

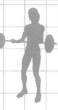

## TIP

Even though you train a lot, showering every day washes away essential natural oils. Rinsing is fine, or showering every other day works too.

# YOUR TRAINING
# JOURNAL

DATE

| EXERCISE | | SET 1 | SET 2 | SET 3 | SET 4 | SET 5 | SET 6 |
|---|---|---|---|---|---|---|---|
| | WEIGHT | | | | | | |
| | REPS | | | | | | |
| | WEIGHT | | | | | | |
| | REPS | | | | | | |
| | WEIGHT | | | | | | |
| | REPS | | | | | | |
| | WEIGHT | | | | | | |
| | REPS | | | | | | |
| | WEIGHT | | | | | | |
| | REPS | | | | | | |
| | WEIGHT | | | | | | |
| | REPS | | | | | | |
| | WEIGHT | | | | | | |
| | REPS | | | | | | |
| | WEIGHT | | | | | | |
| | REPS | | | | | | |
| | WEIGHT | | | | | | |
| | REPS | | | | | | |
| | WEIGHT | | | | | | |
| | REPS | | | | | | |
| | WEIGHT | | | | | | |
| | REPS | | | | | | |

**CARDIO ACTIVITY:**

**NOTES:**

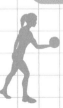

## TIP
An ideal before-training snack or Eat-Clean meal is an apple cut into quarters and spread with natural nut butter. That's complex carb and lean protein fast food!

# YOUR TRAINING
# JOURNAL

DATE

| EXERCISE | | SET 1 | SET 2 | SET 3 | SET 4 | SET 5 | SET 6 |
|---|---|---|---|---|---|---|---|
| | WEIGHT | | | | | | |
| | REPS | | | | | | |
| | WEIGHT | | | | | | |
| | REPS | | | | | | |
| | WEIGHT | | | | | | |
| | REPS | | | | | | |
| | WEIGHT | | | | | | |
| | REPS | | | | | | |
| | WEIGHT | | | | | | |
| | REPS | | | | | | |
| | WEIGHT | | | | | | |
| | REPS | | | | | | |
| | WEIGHT | | | | | | |
| | REPS | | | | | | |
| | WEIGHT | | | | | | |
| | REPS | | | | | | |
| | WEIGHT | | | | | | |
| | REPS | | | | | | |
| | WEIGHT | | | | | | |
| | REPS | | | | | | |
| | WEIGHT | | | | | | |
| | REPS | | | | | | |

**CARDIO ACTIVITY:**

**NOTES:**

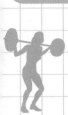

## TIP
Avoid flavored and designer waters. They are often loaded with hidden unwanted ingredients. Toss a few fresh lemon, lime, orange or cucumber slices into your water instead.

# YOUR TRAINING JOURNAL

**DATE** [ ]

| EXERCISE | | SET 1 | SET 2 | SET 3 | SET 4 | SET 5 | SET 6 |
|---|---|---|---|---|---|---|---|
| | WEIGHT | | | | | | |
| | REPS | | | | | | |
| | WEIGHT | | | | | | |
| | REPS | | | | | | |
| | WEIGHT | | | | | | |
| | REPS | | | | | | |
| | WEIGHT | | | | | | |
| | REPS | | | | | | |
| | WEIGHT | | | | | | |
| | REPS | | | | | | |
| | WEIGHT | | | | | | |
| | REPS | | | | | | |
| | WEIGHT | | | | | | |
| | REPS | | | | | | |
| | WEIGHT | | | | | | |
| | REPS | | | | | | |
| | WEIGHT | | | | | | |
| | REPS | | | | | | |
| | WEIGHT | | | | | | |
| | REPS | | | | | | |
| | WEIGHT | | | | | | |
| | REPS | | | | | | |

**CARDIO ACTIVITY:**

**NOTES:**

## TIP

Boil a dozen eggs instead of a few. That way you'll have extras for the next Clean-Eating meal.

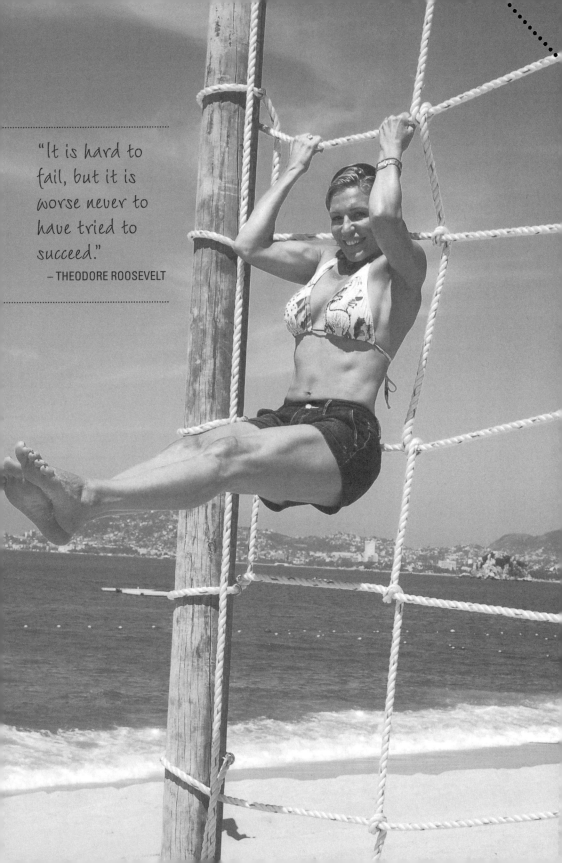

"It is hard to fail, but it is worse never to have tried to succeed."
– THEODORE ROOSEVELT

# YOUR TRAINING
# JOURNAL

**DATE**

| EXERCISE | | SET 1 | SET 2 | SET 3 | SET 4 | SET 5 | SET 6 |
|---|---|---|---|---|---|---|---|
| | WEIGHT | | | | | | |
| | REPS | | | | | | |
| | WEIGHT | | | | | | |
| | REPS | | | | | | |
| | WEIGHT | | | | | | |
| | REPS | | | | | | |
| | WEIGHT | | | | | | |
| | REPS | | | | | | |
| | WEIGHT | | | | | | |
| | REPS | | | | | | |
| | WEIGHT | | | | | | |
| | REPS | | | | | | |
| | WEIGHT | | | | | | |
| | REPS | | | | | | |
| | WEIGHT | | | | | | |
| | REPS | | | | | | |
| | WEIGHT | | | | | | |
| | REPS | | | | | | |
| | WEIGHT | | | | | | |
| | REPS | | | | | | |
| | WEIGHT | | | | | | |
| | REPS | | | | | | |

**CARDIO ACTIVITY:**

**NOTES:**

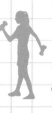

## TIP

Keep your cooler handy and prepped with small jars of natural nut butters, raw unsalted nuts, apples and plain oatmeal. With these ingredients already packed, the rest is simple.

# YOUR TRAINING JOURNAL

**DATE**

| EXERCISE | | SET 1 | SET 2 | SET 3 | SET 4 | SET 5 | SET 6 |
|---|---|---|---|---|---|---|---|
| | WEIGHT | | | | | | |
| | REPS | | | | | | |
| | WEIGHT | | | | | | |
| | REPS | | | | | | |
| | WEIGHT | | | | | | |
| | REPS | | | | | | |
| | WEIGHT | | | | | | |
| | REPS | | | | | | |
| | WEIGHT | | | | | | |
| | REPS | | | | | | |
| | WEIGHT | | | | | | |
| | REPS | | | | | | |
| | WEIGHT | | | | | | |
| | REPS | | | | | | |
| | WEIGHT | | | | | | |
| | REPS | | | | | | |
| | WEIGHT | | | | | | |
| | REPS | | | | | | |
| | WEIGHT | | | | | | |
| | REPS | | | | | | |
| | WEIGHT | | | | | | |
| | REPS | | | | | | |

**CARDIO ACTIVITY:**

**NOTES:**

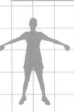

## TIP
Load your iPod with energized music. A good tune will get you through any workout.

# YOUR TRAINING
# JOURNAL

DATE

| EXERCISE | | SET 1 | SET 2 | SET 3 | SET 4 | SET 5 | SET 6 |
|---|---|---|---|---|---|---|---|
| | WEIGHT | | | | | | |
| | REPS | | | | | | |
| | WEIGHT | | | | | | |
| | REPS | | | | | | |
| | WEIGHT | | | | | | |
| | REPS | | | | | | |
| | WEIGHT | | | | | | |
| | REPS | | | | | | |
| | WEIGHT | | | | | | |
| | REPS | | | | | | |
| | WEIGHT | | | | | | |
| | REPS | | | | | | |
| | WEIGHT | | | | | | |
| | REPS | | | | | | |
| | WEIGHT | | | | | | |
| | REPS | | | | | | |
| | WEIGHT | | | | | | |
| | REPS | | | | | | |
| | WEIGHT | | | | | | |
| | REPS | | | | | | |
| | WEIGHT | | | | | | |
| | REPS | | | | | | |

**CARDIO ACTIVITY:**

**NOTES:**

## TIP

Train with a partner to help motivate you and to learn new training tips.

# YOUR TRAINING JOURNAL

**DATE**

| EXERCISE | | SET 1 | SET 2 | SET 3 | SET 4 | SET 5 | SET 6 |
|---|---|---|---|---|---|---|---|
| | WEIGHT | | | | | | |
| | REPS | | | | | | |
| | WEIGHT | | | | | | |
| | REPS | | | | | | |
| | WEIGHT | | | | | | |
| | REPS | | | | | | |
| | WEIGHT | | | | | | |
| | REPS | | | | | | |
| | WEIGHT | | | | | | |
| | REPS | | | | | | |
| | WEIGHT | | | | | | |
| | REPS | | | | | | |
| | WEIGHT | | | | | | |
| | REPS | | | | | | |
| | WEIGHT | | | | | | |
| | REPS | | | | | | |
| | WEIGHT | | | | | | |
| | REPS | | | | | | |
| | WEIGHT | | | | | | |
| | REPS | | | | | | |
| | WEIGHT | | | | | | |
| | REPS | | | | | | |

**CARDIO ACTIVITY:**

**NOTES:**

**TIP**

Attend a training boot camp to put a new spin on your workouts.

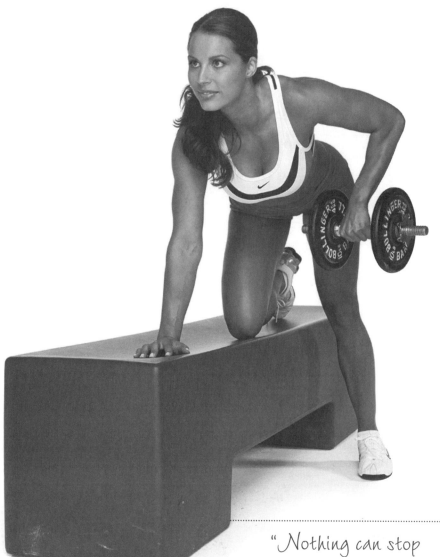

" Nothing can stop
someone with the right
mental attitude from
achieving his or her goal;
nothing on earth can help
the person with the wrong
mental attitude."

– THOMAS JEFFERSON

# YOUR TRAINING JOURNAL

DATE

| EXERCISE | | SET 1 | SET 2 | SET 3 | SET 4 | SET 5 | SET 6 |
|---|---|---|---|---|---|---|---|
| | WEIGHT | | | | | | |
| | REPS | | | | | | |
| | WEIGHT | | | | | | |
| | REPS | | | | | | |
| | WEIGHT | | | | | | |
| | REPS | | | | | | |
| | WEIGHT | | | | | | |
| | REPS | | | | | | |
| | WEIGHT | | | | | | |
| | REPS | | | | | | |
| | WEIGHT | | | | | | |
| | REPS | | | | | | |
| | WEIGHT | | | | | | |
| | REPS | | | | | | |
| | WEIGHT | | | | | | |
| | REPS | | | | | | |
| | WEIGHT | | | | | | |
| | REPS | | | | | | |
| | WEIGHT | | | | | | |
| | REPS | | | | | | |
| | WEIGHT | | | | | | |
| | REPS | | | | | | |

**CARDIO ACTIVITY:**

**NOTES:**

## TIP
Need a blitz to eliminate flabby upper arms? Alternate two triceps exercises without stopping for 4 sets of 12 reps each.

# YOUR TRAINING
# JOURNAL

DATE

| EXERCISE | | SET 1 | SET 2 | SET 3 | SET 4 | SET 5 | SET 6 |
|----------|-----|-------|-------|-------|-------|-------|-------|
| | WEIGHT | | | | | | |
| | REPS | | | | | | |
| | WEIGHT | | | | | | |
| | REPS | | | | | | |
| | WEIGHT | | | | | | |
| | REPS | | | | | | |
| | WEIGHT | | | | | | |
| | REPS | | | | | | |
| | WEIGHT | | | | | | |
| | REPS | | | | | | |
| | WEIGHT | | | | | | |
| | REPS | | | | | | |
| | WEIGHT | | | | | | |
| | REPS | | | | | | |
| | WEIGHT | | | | | | |
| | REPS | | | | | | |
| | WEIGHT | | | | | | |
| | REPS | | | | | | |
| | WEIGHT | | | | | | |
| | REPS | | | | | | |
| | WEIGHT | | | | | | |
| | REPS | | | | | | |

**CARDIO ACTIVITY:**

**NOTES:**

## TIP
Want strength without additional size? Use 4 reps per set and keep food intake lean.

# YOUR TRAINING JOURNAL

DATE

| EXERCISE | | SET 1 | SET 2 | SET 3 | SET 4 | SET 5 | SET 6 |
|---|---|---|---|---|---|---|---|
| | WEIGHT | | | | | | |
| | REPS | | | | | | |
| | WEIGHT | | | | | | |
| | REPS | | | | | | |
| | WEIGHT | | | | | | |
| | REPS | | | | | | |
| | WEIGHT | | | | | | |
| | REPS | | | | | | |
| | WEIGHT | | | | | | |
| | REPS | | | | | | |
| | WEIGHT | | | | | | |
| | REPS | | | | | | |
| | WEIGHT | | | | | | |
| | REPS | | | | | | |
| | WEIGHT | | | | | | |
| | REPS | | | | | | |
| | WEIGHT | | | | | | |
| | REPS | | | | | | |
| | WEIGHT | | | | | | |
| | REPS | | | | | | |
| | WEIGHT | | | | | | |
| | REPS | | | | | | |

**CARDIO ACTIVITY:**

**NOTES:**

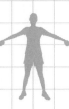

## TIP

When you start twisting the shoulders, arms and body to get a weight moving, you have lost form. Stop the set immediately.

# YOUR TRAINING
# JOURNAL

DATE

| EXERCISE | | SET 1 | SET 2 | SET 3 | SET 4 | SET 5 | SET 6 |
|---|---|---|---|---|---|---|---|
| | WEIGHT | | | | | | |
| | REPS | | | | | | |
| | WEIGHT | | | | | | |
| | REPS | | | | | | |
| | WEIGHT | | | | | | |
| | REPS | | | | | | |
| | WEIGHT | | | | | | |
| | REPS | | | | | | |
| | WEIGHT | | | | | | |
| | REPS | | | | | | |
| | WEIGHT | | | | | | |
| | REPS | | | | | | |
| | WEIGHT | | | | | | |
| | REPS | | | | | | |
| | WEIGHT | | | | | | |
| | REPS | | | | | | |
| | WEIGHT | | | | | | |
| | REPS | | | | | | |
| | WEIGHT | | | | | | |
| | REPS | | | | | | |
| | WEIGHT | | | | | | |
| | REPS | | | | | | |

**CARDIO ACTIVITY:**

**NOTES:**

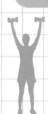

## TIP
If your body is feeling constantly exhausted and your enthusiasm for training is waning, take a whole week off.

# YOUR TRAINING
# JOURNAL

**DATE**

| EXERCISE | | SET 1 | SET 2 | SET 3 | SET 4 | SET 5 | SET 6 |
|---|---|---|---|---|---|---|---|
| | WEIGHT | | | | | | |
| | REPS | | | | | | |
| | WEIGHT | | | | | | |
| | REPS | | | | | | |
| | WEIGHT | | | | | | |
| | REPS | | | | | | |
| | WEIGHT | | | | | | |
| | REPS | | | | | | |
| | WEIGHT | | | | | | |
| | REPS | | | | | | |
| | WEIGHT | | | | | | |
| | REPS | | | | | | |
| | WEIGHT | | | | | | |
| | REPS | | | | | | |
| | WEIGHT | | | | | | |
| | REPS | | | | | | |
| | WEIGHT | | | | | | |
| | REPS | | | | | | |
| | WEIGHT | | | | | | |
| | REPS | | | | | | |
| | WEIGHT | | | | | | |
| | REPS | | | | | | |

**CARDIO ACTIVITY:**

**NOTES:**

## TIP
Short of time? Don't perform one-leg or one-arm exercises. Work both sides together.

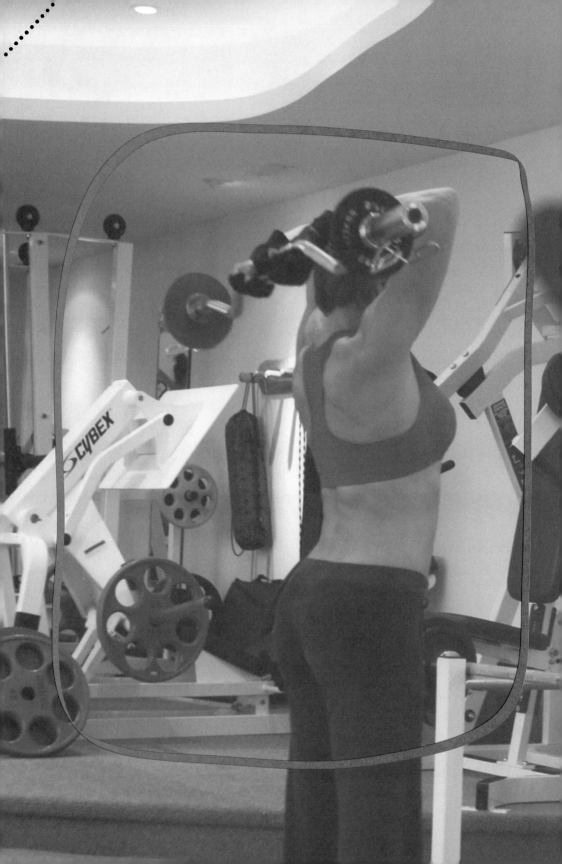

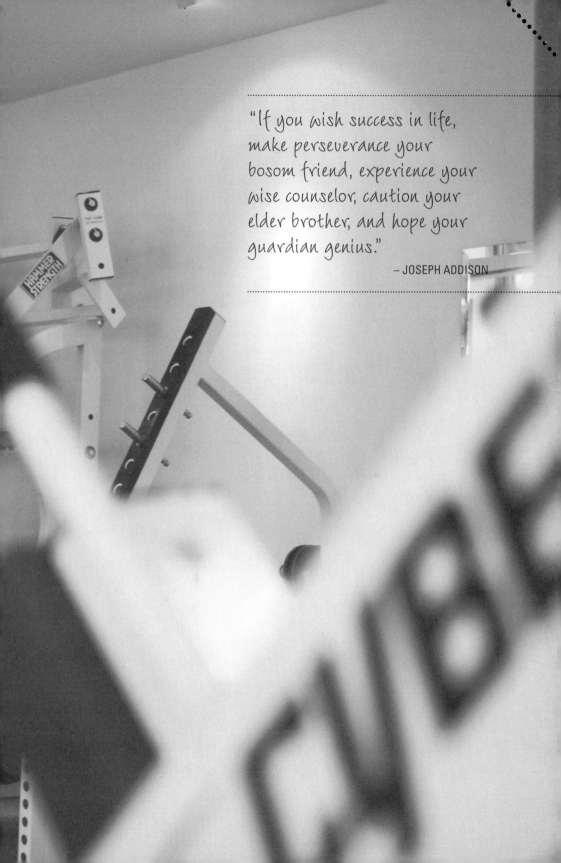

"If you wish success in life, make perseverance your bosom friend, experience your wise counselor, caution your elder brother, and hope your guardian genius."

– JOSEPH ADDISON

# YOUR TRAINING
# JOURNAL

DATE

| EXERCISE | | SET 1 | SET 2 | SET 3 | SET 4 | SET 5 | SET 6 |
|---|---|---|---|---|---|---|---|
| | WEIGHT | | | | | | |
| | REPS | | | | | | |
| | WEIGHT | | | | | | |
| | REPS | | | | | | |
| | WEIGHT | | | | | | |
| | REPS | | | | | | |
| | WEIGHT | | | | | | |
| | REPS | | | | | | |
| | WEIGHT | | | | | | |
| | REPS | | | | | | |
| | WEIGHT | | | | | | |
| | REPS | | | | | | |
| | WEIGHT | | | | | | |
| | REPS | | | | | | |
| | WEIGHT | | | | | | |
| | REPS | | | | | | |
| | WEIGHT | | | | | | |
| | REPS | | | | | | |
| | WEIGHT | | | | | | |
| | REPS | | | | | | |
| | WEIGHT | | | | | | |
| | REPS | | | | | | |

**CARDIO ACTIVITY:**

**NOTES:**

## TIP
The question of drinking: A glass of wine a day can be
beneficial but cut out all alcohol when going for peak condition.

# YOUR TRAINING
# JOURNAL

**DATE**

| EXERCISE | | SET 1 | SET 2 | SET 3 | SET 4 | SET 5 | SET 6 |
|---|---|---|---|---|---|---|---|
| | WEIGHT | | | | | | |
| | REPS | | | | | | |
| | WEIGHT | | | | | | |
| | REPS | | | | | | |
| | WEIGHT | | | | | | |
| | REPS | | | | | | |
| | WEIGHT | | | | | | |
| | REPS | | | | | | |
| | WEIGHT | | | | | | |
| | REPS | | | | | | |
| | WEIGHT | | | | | | |
| | REPS | | | | | | |
| | WEIGHT | | | | | | |
| | REPS | | | | | | |
| | WEIGHT | | | | | | |
| | REPS | | | | | | |
| | WEIGHT | | | | | | |
| | REPS | | | | | | |
| | WEIGHT | | | | | | |
| | REPS | | | | | | |
| | WEIGHT | | | | | | |
| | REPS | | | | | | |

**CARDIO ACTIVITY:**

**NOTES:**

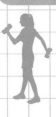

## TIP
Coffee and tea are mild diuretics, but stay away from
diuretic drugs.

# YOUR TRAINING JOURNAL

**DATE**

| EXERCISE | | SET 1 | SET 2 | SET 3 | SET 4 | SET 5 | SET 6 |
|---|---|---|---|---|---|---|---|
| | WEIGHT | | | | | | |
| | REPS | | | | | | |
| | WEIGHT | | | | | | |
| | REPS | | | | | | |
| | WEIGHT | | | | | | |
| | REPS | | | | | | |
| | WEIGHT | | | | | | |
| | REPS | | | | | | |
| | WEIGHT | | | | | | |
| | REPS | | | | | | |
| | WEIGHT | | | | | | |
| | REPS | | | | | | |
| | WEIGHT | | | | | | |
| | REPS | | | | | | |
| | WEIGHT | | | | | | |
| | REPS | | | | | | |
| | WEIGHT | | | | | | |
| | REPS | | | | | | |
| | WEIGHT | | | | | | |
| | REPS | | | | | | |
| | WEIGHT | | | | | | |
| | REPS | | | | | | |

**CARDIO ACTIVITY:**

**NOTES:**

## TIP

Decrease your rest periods between exercises when aiming for fat loss. More work in less time is another way of increasing intensity.

# YOUR TRAINING JOURNAL

DATE

| EXERCISE | | SET 1 | SET 2 | SET 3 | SET 4 | SET 5 | SET 6 |
|---|---|---|---|---|---|---|---|
| | WEIGHT | | | | | | |
| | REPS | | | | | | |
| | WEIGHT | | | | | | |
| | REPS | | | | | | |
| | WEIGHT | | | | | | |
| | REPS | | | | | | |
| | WEIGHT | | | | | | |
| | REPS | | | | | | |
| | WEIGHT | | | | | | |
| | REPS | | | | | | |
| | WEIGHT | | | | | | |
| | REPS | | | | | | |
| | WEIGHT | | | | | | |
| | REPS | | | | | | |
| | WEIGHT | | | | | | |
| | REPS | | | | | | |
| | WEIGHT | | | | | | |
| | REPS | | | | | | |
| | WEIGHT | | | | | | |
| | REPS | | | | | | |
| | WEIGHT | | | | | | |
| | REPS | | | | | | |

**CARDIO ACTIVITY:**

**NOTES:**

**TIP**
Don't waste time counting calories. The counts are never accurate, and it's the garbage in foods that make us fat, not necessarily the calorie total.

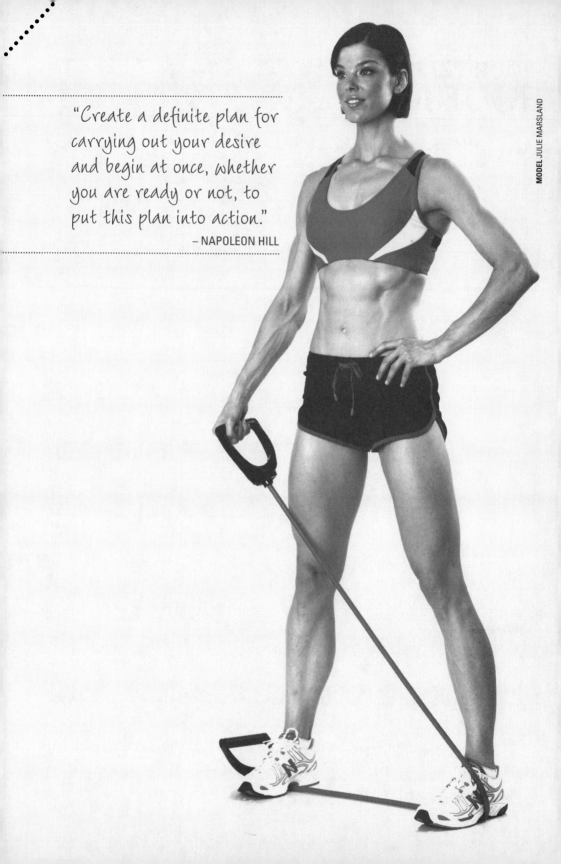

"Create a definite plan for carrying out your desire and begin at once, whether you are ready or not, to put this plan into action."

– NAPOLEON HILL

# YOUR TRAINING JOURNAL

DATE

| EXERCISE | | SET 1 | SET 2 | SET 3 | SET 4 | SET 5 | SET 6 |
|---|---|---|---|---|---|---|---|
| | WEIGHT | | | | | | |
| | REPS | | | | | | |
| | WEIGHT | | | | | | |
| | REPS | | | | | | |
| | WEIGHT | | | | | | |
| | REPS | | | | | | |
| | WEIGHT | | | | | | |
| | REPS | | | | | | |
| | WEIGHT | | | | | | |
| | REPS | | | | | | |
| | WEIGHT | | | | | | |
| | REPS | | | | | | |
| | WEIGHT | | | | | | |
| | REPS | | | | | | |
| | WEIGHT | | | | | | |
| | REPS | | | | | | |
| | WEIGHT | | | | | | |
| | REPS | | | | | | |
| | WEIGHT | | | | | | |
| | REPS | | | | | | |
| | WEIGHT | | | | | | |
| | REPS | | | | | | |

**CARDIO ACTIVITY:**

**NOTES:**

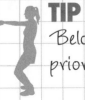

## TIP
Below-standard calves? Stretch for six to eight minutes prior to your heavy-resistance calf exercises.

# YOUR TRAINING JOURNAL

DATE

| EXERCISE | | SET 1 | SET 2 | SET 3 | SET 4 | SET 5 | SET 6 |
|---|---|---|---|---|---|---|---|
| | WEIGHT | | | | | | |
| | REPS | | | | | | |
| | WEIGHT | | | | | | |
| | REPS | | | | | | |
| | WEIGHT | | | | | | |
| | REPS | | | | | | |
| | WEIGHT | | | | | | |
| | REPS | | | | | | |
| | WEIGHT | | | | | | |
| | REPS | | | | | | |
| | WEIGHT | | | | | | |
| | REPS | | | | | | |
| | WEIGHT | | | | | | |
| | REPS | | | | | | |
| | WEIGHT | | | | | | |
| | REPS | | | | | | |
| | WEIGHT | | | | | | |
| | REPS | | | | | | |
| | WEIGHT | | | | | | |
| | REPS | | | | | | |
| | WEIGHT | | | | | | |
| | REPS | | | | | | |

**CARDIO ACTIVITY:**

**NOTES:**

## TIP

Poor shoulders? Use Robert Kennedy's pre-exhaust system. Ten reps of barbell upright rows alternated with 10 reps of barbell shoulder presses. Three sets of each.

# YOUR TRAINING JOURNAL

DATE

| EXERCISE | | SET 1 | SET 2 | SET 3 | SET 4 | SET 5 | SET 6 |
|---|---|---|---|---|---|---|---|
| | WEIGHT | | | | | | |
| | REPS | | | | | | |
| | WEIGHT | | | | | | |
| | REPS | | | | | | |
| | WEIGHT | | | | | | |
| | REPS | | | | | | |
| | WEIGHT | | | | | | |
| | REPS | | | | | | |
| | WEIGHT | | | | | | |
| | REPS | | | | | | |
| | WEIGHT | | | | | | |
| | REPS | | | | | | |
| | WEIGHT | | | | | | |
| | REPS | | | | | | |
| | WEIGHT | | | | | | |
| | REPS | | | | | | |
| | WEIGHT | | | | | | |
| | REPS | | | | | | |
| | WEIGHT | | | | | | |
| | REPS | | | | | | |
| | WEIGHT | | | | | | |
| | REPS | | | | | | |

**CARDIO ACTIVITY:**

**NOTES:**

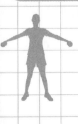

## TIP

Eat for energy — muesli, oatmeal, sweet potatoes, fruit, brown rice — before your workout. Eat for muscle repair — meat, fish, poultry, egg whites, nuts, soy, legumes — after your workout.

# YOUR TRAINING
# JOURNAL

DATE

| EXERCISE | | SET 1 | SET 2 | SET 3 | SET 4 | SET 5 | SET 6 |
|---|---|---|---|---|---|---|---|
| | WEIGHT | | | | | | |
| | REPS | | | | | | |
| | WEIGHT | | | | | | |
| | REPS | | | | | | |
| | WEIGHT | | | | | | |
| | REPS | | | | | | |
| | WEIGHT | | | | | | |
| | REPS | | | | | | |
| | WEIGHT | | | | | | |
| | REPS | | | | | | |
| | WEIGHT | | | | | | |
| | REPS | | | | | | |
| | WEIGHT | | | | | | |
| | REPS | | | | | | |
| | WEIGHT | | | | | | |
| | REPS | | | | | | |
| | WEIGHT | | | | | | |
| | REPS | | | | | | |
| | WEIGHT | | | | | | |
| | REPS | | | | | | |
| | WEIGHT | | | | | | |
| | REPS | | | | | | |

**CARDIO ACTIVITY:**

**NOTES:**

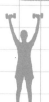

**TIP**

If your wrists hurt during some exercises, consider using an EZ-Curl bar for added comfort.

# YOUR TRAINING
# JOURNAL

**DATE**

| EXERCISE | | SET 1 | SET 2 | SET 3 | SET 4 | SET 5 | SET 6 |
|---|---|---|---|---|---|---|---|
| | WEIGHT | | | | | | |
| | REPS | | | | | | |
| | WEIGHT | | | | | | |
| | REPS | | | | | | |
| | WEIGHT | | | | | | |
| | REPS | | | | | | |
| | WEIGHT | | | | | | |
| | REPS | | | | | | |
| | WEIGHT | | | | | | |
| | REPS | | | | | | |
| | WEIGHT | | | | | | |
| | REPS | | | | | | |
| | WEIGHT | | | | | | |
| | REPS | | | | | | |
| | WEIGHT | | | | | | |
| | REPS | | | | | | |
| | WEIGHT | | | | | | |
| | REPS | | | | | | |
| | WEIGHT | | | | | | |
| | REPS | | | | | | |
| | WEIGHT | | | | | | |
| | REPS | | | | | | |

**CARDIO ACTIVITY:**

**NOTES:**

## TIP
Don't bounce the weight on your chest during the bench press.

# YOUR TRAINING JOURNAL

DATE

| EXERCISE | | SET 1 | SET 2 | SET 3 | SET 4 | SET 5 | SET 6 |
|---|---|---|---|---|---|---|---|
| | WEIGHT | | | | | | |
| | REPS | | | | | | |
| | WEIGHT | | | | | | |
| | REPS | | | | | | |
| | WEIGHT | | | | | | |
| | REPS | | | | | | |
| | WEIGHT | | | | | | |
| | REPS | | | | | | |
| | WEIGHT | | | | | | |
| | REPS | | | | | | |
| | WEIGHT | | | | | | |
| | REPS | | | | | | |
| | WEIGHT | | | | | | |
| | REPS | | | | | | |
| | WEIGHT | | | | | | |
| | REPS | | | | | | |
| | WEIGHT | | | | | | |
| | REPS | | | | | | |
| | WEIGHT | | | | | | |
| | REPS | | | | | | |
| | WEIGHT | | | | | | |
| | REPS | | | | | | |

**CARDIO ACTIVITY:**

**NOTES:**

## TIP
Don't try the following exercises on a fitball: squats, bench presses, lunges, or any exercise that obviously invites a precarious accident.

# YOUR TRAINING JOURNAL

**DATE**

| EXERCISE | | SET 1 | SET 2 | SET 3 | SET 4 | SET 5 | SET 6 |
|---|---|---|---|---|---|---|---|
| | WEIGHT | | | | | | |
| | REPS | | | | | | |
| | WEIGHT | | | | | | |
| | REPS | | | | | | |
| | WEIGHT | | | | | | |
| | REPS | | | | | | |
| | WEIGHT | | | | | | |
| | REPS | | | | | | |
| | WEIGHT | | | | | | |
| | REPS | | | | | | |
| | WEIGHT | | | | | | |
| | REPS | | | | | | |
| | WEIGHT | | | | | | |
| | REPS | | | | | | |
| | WEIGHT | | | | | | |
| | REPS | | | | | | |
| | WEIGHT | | | | | | |
| | REPS | | | | | | |
| | WEIGHT | | | | | | |
| | REPS | | | | | | |
| | WEIGHT | | | | | | |
| | REPS | | | | | | |

**CARDIO ACTIVITY:**

**NOTES:**

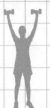

## TIP

When performing incline chest work — presses or flyes — place the bench at a 30- to 35-degree angle, not at the standard 45- to 50-degree angle.

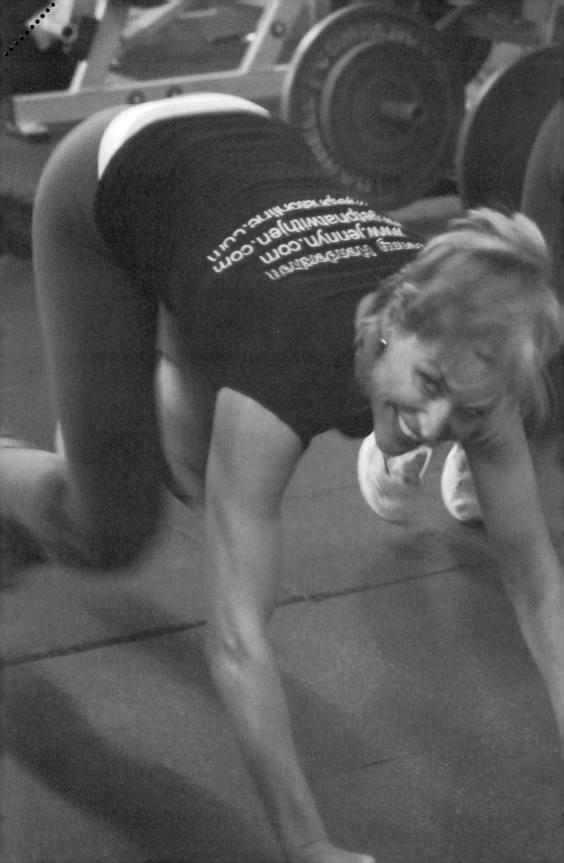

"Success is the good fortune that comes from aspiration, desperation, perspiration and inspiration."

— EVAN ESAR

# YOUR TRAINING
# JOURNAL

DATE

| EXERCISE | | SET 1 | SET 2 | SET 3 | SET 4 | SET 5 | SET 6 |
|---|---|---|---|---|---|---|---|
| | WEIGHT | | | | | | |
| | REPS | | | | | | |
| | WEIGHT | | | | | | |
| | REPS | | | | | | |
| | WEIGHT | | | | | | |
| | REPS | | | | | | |
| | WEIGHT | | | | | | |
| | REPS | | | | | | |
| | WEIGHT | | | | | | |
| | REPS | | | | | | |
| | WEIGHT | | | | | | |
| | REPS | | | | | | |
| | WEIGHT | | | | | | |
| | REPS | | | | | | |
| | WEIGHT | | | | | | |
| | REPS | | | | | | |
| | WEIGHT | | | | | | |
| | REPS | | | | | | |
| | WEIGHT | | | | | | |
| | REPS | | | | | | |
| | WEIGHT | | | | | | |
| | REPS | | | | | | |

**CARDIO ACTIVITY:**

**NOTES:**

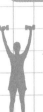

## TIP

A whole-body warmup using the treadmill, running in place, or rope jumping is a good idea before starting your weight- training routine. A few minutes will get your blood circulating and your heart pumping for further action.

# YOUR TRAINING JOURNAL

**DATE**

| EXERCISE | | SET 1 | SET 2 | SET 3 | SET 4 | SET 5 | SET 6 |
|---|---|---|---|---|---|---|---|
| | WEIGHT | | | | | | |
| | REPS | | | | | | |
| | WEIGHT | | | | | | |
| | REPS | | | | | | |
| | WEIGHT | | | | | | |
| | REPS | | | | | | |
| | WEIGHT | | | | | | |
| | REPS | | | | | | |
| | WEIGHT | | | | | | |
| | REPS | | | | | | |
| | WEIGHT | | | | | | |
| | REPS | | | | | | |
| | WEIGHT | | | | | | |
| | REPS | | | | | | |
| | WEIGHT | | | | | | |
| | REPS | | | | | | |
| | WEIGHT | | | | | | |
| | REPS | | | | | | |
| | WEIGHT | | | | | | |
| | REPS | | | | | | |
| | WEIGHT | | | | | | |
| | REPS | | | | | | |

**CARDIO ACTIVITY:**

**NOTES:**

**TIP**

Make your rep counting easier. Count in groups of four.

# YOUR TRAINING
# JOURNAL

**DATE** [ ]

| EXERCISE | | SET 1 | SET 2 | SET 3 | SET 4 | SET 5 | SET 6 |
|---|---|---|---|---|---|---|---|
| | WEIGHT | | | | | | |
| | REPS | | | | | | |
| | WEIGHT | | | | | | |
| | REPS | | | | | | |
| | WEIGHT | | | | | | |
| | REPS | | | | | | |
| | WEIGHT | | | | | | |
| | REPS | | | | | | |
| | WEIGHT | | | | | | |
| | REPS | | | | | | |
| | WEIGHT | | | | | | |
| | REPS | | | | | | |
| | WEIGHT | | | | | | |
| | REPS | | | | | | |
| | WEIGHT | | | | | | |
| | REPS | | | | | | |
| | WEIGHT | | | | | | |
| | REPS | | | | | | |
| | WEIGHT | | | | | | |
| | REPS | | | | | | |
| | WEIGHT | | | | | | |
| | REPS | | | | | | |

**CARDIO ACTIVITY:**

**NOTES:**

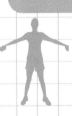

## TIP
Begin your workouts by training your weakest
body part first.

# YOUR TRAINING
# JOURNAL

DATE

| EXERCISE | | SET 1 | SET 2 | SET 3 | SET 4 | SET 5 | SET 6 |
|---|---|---|---|---|---|---|---|
| | WEIGHT | | | | | | |
| | REPS | | | | | | |
| | WEIGHT | | | | | | |
| | REPS | | | | | | |
| | WEIGHT | | | | | | |
| | REPS | | | | | | |
| | WEIGHT | | | | | | |
| | REPS | | | | | | |
| | WEIGHT | | | | | | |
| | REPS | | | | | | |
| | WEIGHT | | | | | | |
| | REPS | | | | | | |
| | WEIGHT | | | | | | |
| | REPS | | | | | | |
| | WEIGHT | | | | | | |
| | REPS | | | | | | |
| | WEIGHT | | | | | | |
| | REPS | | | | | | |
| | WEIGHT | | | | | | |
| | REPS | | | | | | |
| | WEIGHT | | | | | | |
| | REPS | | | | | | |

**CARDIO ACTIVITY:**

**NOTES:**

## TIP
Eat six small meals a day for best results.

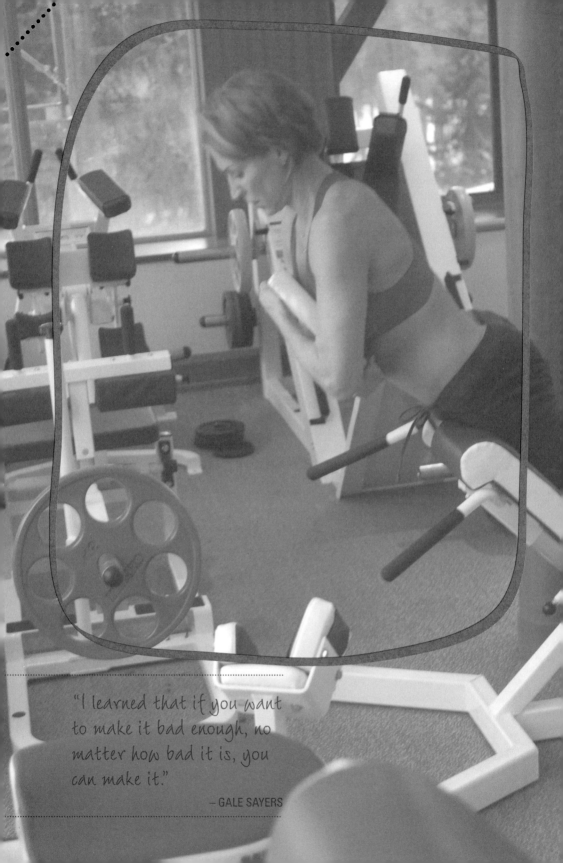

"I learned that if you want to make it bad enough, no matter how bad it is, you can make it."

— GALE SAYERS

# YOUR TRAINING JOURNAL

DATE

| EXERCISE | | SET 1 | SET 2 | SET 3 | SET 4 | SET 5 | SET 6 |
|---|---|---|---|---|---|---|---|
| | WEIGHT | | | | | | |
| | REPS | | | | | | |
| | WEIGHT | | | | | | |
| | REPS | | | | | | |
| | WEIGHT | | | | | | |
| | REPS | | | | | | |
| | WEIGHT | | | | | | |
| | REPS | | | | | | |
| | WEIGHT | | | | | | |
| | REPS | | | | | | |
| | WEIGHT | | | | | | |
| | REPS | | | | | | |
| | WEIGHT | | | | | | |
| | REPS | | | | | | |
| | WEIGHT | | | | | | |
| | REPS | | | | | | |
| | WEIGHT | | | | | | |
| | REPS | | | | | | |
| | WEIGHT | | | | | | |
| | REPS | | | | | | |
| | WEIGHT | | | | | | |
| | REPS | | | | | | |

**CARDIO ACTIVITY:**

**NOTES:**

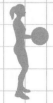

**TIP**
Put your mind into the muscle. Think about the body part you are challenging.

# YOUR TRAINING JOURNAL

**DATE**

| EXERCISE | | SET 1 | SET 2 | SET 3 | SET 4 | SET 5 | SET 6 |
|---|---|---|---|---|---|---|---|
| | WEIGHT | | | | | | |
| | REPS | | | | | | |
| | WEIGHT | | | | | | |
| | REPS | | | | | | |
| | WEIGHT | | | | | | |
| | REPS | | | | | | |
| | WEIGHT | | | | | | |
| | REPS | | | | | | |
| | WEIGHT | | | | | | |
| | REPS | | | | | | |
| | WEIGHT | | | | | | |
| | REPS | | | | | | |
| | WEIGHT | | | | | | |
| | REPS | | | | | | |
| | WEIGHT | | | | | | |
| | REPS | | | | | | |
| | WEIGHT | | | | | | |
| | REPS | | | | | | |
| | WEIGHT | | | | | | |
| | REPS | | | | | | |
| | WEIGHT | | | | | | |
| | REPS | | | | | | |

**CARDIO ACTIVITY:**

**NOTES:**

## TIP

If you don't know how, learn how to cook basic Clean-Eating foods including oatmeal, fish, steamed veggies and chicken breasts.

# YOUR TRAINING JOURNAL

**DATE**

| EXERCISE | | SET 1 | SET 2 | SET 3 | SET 4 | SET 5 | SET 6 |
|---|---|---|---|---|---|---|---|
| | WEIGHT | | | | | | |
| | REPS | | | | | | |
| | WEIGHT | | | | | | |
| | REPS | | | | | | |
| | WEIGHT | | | | | | |
| | REPS | | | | | | |
| | WEIGHT | | | | | | |
| | REPS | | | | | | |
| | WEIGHT | | | | | | |
| | REPS | | | | | | |
| | WEIGHT | | | | | | |
| | REPS | | | | | | |
| | WEIGHT | | | | | | |
| | REPS | | | | | | |
| | WEIGHT | | | | | | |
| | REPS | | | | | | |
| | WEIGHT | | | | | | |
| | REPS | | | | | | |
| | WEIGHT | | | | | | |
| | REPS | | | | | | |
| | WEIGHT | | | | | | |
| | REPS | | | | | | |

**CARDIO ACTIVITY:**

**NOTES:**

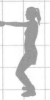

## TIP
Perform leg work on the hack machine if you want to improve the outer sweep of your quads.

# YOUR TRAINING JOURNAL

**DATE**

| EXERCISE | | SET 1 | SET 2 | SET 3 | SET 4 | SET 5 | SET 6 |
|---|---|---|---|---|---|---|---|
| | WEIGHT | | | | | | |
| | REPS | | | | | | |
| | WEIGHT | | | | | | |
| | REPS | | | | | | |
| | WEIGHT | | | | | | |
| | REPS | | | | | | |
| | WEIGHT | | | | | | |
| | REPS | | | | | | |
| | WEIGHT | | | | | | |
| | REPS | | | | | | |
| | WEIGHT | | | | | | |
| | REPS | | | | | | |
| | WEIGHT | | | | | | |
| | REPS | | | | | | |
| | WEIGHT | | | | | | |
| | REPS | | | | | | |
| | WEIGHT | | | | | | |
| | REPS | | | | | | |
| | WEIGHT | | | | | | |
| | REPS | | | | | | |
| | WEIGHT | | | | | | |
| | REPS | | | | | | |

**CARDIO ACTIVITY:**

**NOTES:**

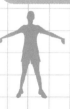

## TIP
Take regular photos of yourself so you can see how you are progressing.

# YOUR TRAINING JOURNAL

**DATE**

| EXERCISE | | SET 1 | SET 2 | SET 3 | SET 4 | SET 5 | SET 6 |
|---|---|---|---|---|---|---|---|
| | WEIGHT | | | | | | |
| | REPS | | | | | | |
| | WEIGHT | | | | | | |
| | REPS | | | | | | |
| | WEIGHT | | | | | | |
| | REPS | | | | | | |
| | WEIGHT | | | | | | |
| | REPS | | | | | | |
| | WEIGHT | | | | | | |
| | REPS | | | | | | |
| | WEIGHT | | | | | | |
| | REPS | | | | | | |
| | WEIGHT | | | | | | |
| | REPS | | | | | | |
| | WEIGHT | | | | | | |
| | REPS | | | | | | |
| | WEIGHT | | | | | | |
| | REPS | | | | | | |
| | WEIGHT | | | | | | |
| | REPS | | | | | | |
| | WEIGHT | | | | | | |
| | REPS | | | | | | |

**CARDIO ACTIVITY:**

**NOTES:**

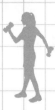

## TIP

Get out of the habit of eating at fast-food establishments.

# YOUR TRAINING
# JOURNAL

**DATE**

| EXERCISE | | SET 1 | SET 2 | SET 3 | SET 4 | SET 5 | SET 6 |
|---|---|---|---|---|---|---|---|
| | WEIGHT | | | | | | |
| | REPS | | | | | | |
| | WEIGHT | | | | | | |
| | REPS | | | | | | |
| | WEIGHT | | | | | | |
| | REPS | | | | | | |
| | WEIGHT | | | | | | |
| | REPS | | | | | | |
| | WEIGHT | | | | | | |
| | REPS | | | | | | |
| | WEIGHT | | | | | | |
| | REPS | | | | | | |
| | WEIGHT | | | | | | |
| | REPS | | | | | | |
| | WEIGHT | | | | | | |
| | REPS | | | | | | |
| | WEIGHT | | | | | | |
| | REPS | | | | | | |
| | WEIGHT | | | | | | |
| | REPS | | | | | | |
| | WEIGHT | | | | | | |
| | REPS | | | | | | |

**CARDIO ACTIVITY:**

**NOTES:**

## TIP
Forget the scales. Go by your mirror image, but look with a critical eye.

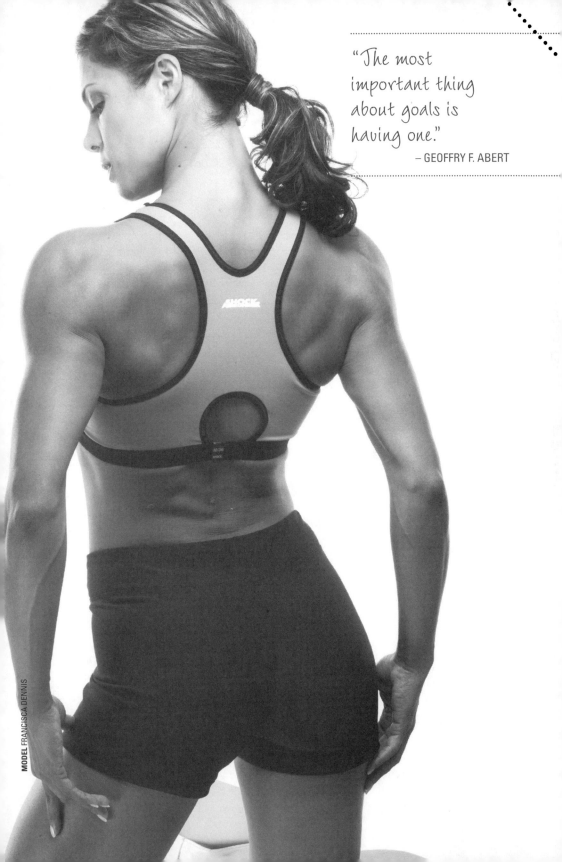

"The most important thing about goals is having one."
– GEOFFRY F. ABERT

MODEL FRANCISCA DENNIS

# YOUR TRAINING
# JOURNAL

**DATE**

| EXERCISE | | SET 1 | SET 2 | SET 3 | SET 4 | SET 5 | SET 6 |
|---|---|---|---|---|---|---|---|
| | WEIGHT | | | | | | |
| | REPS | | | | | | |
| | WEIGHT | | | | | | |
| | REPS | | | | | | |
| | WEIGHT | | | | | | |
| | REPS | | | | | | |
| | WEIGHT | | | | | | |
| | REPS | | | | | | |
| | WEIGHT | | | | | | |
| | REPS | | | | | | |
| | WEIGHT | | | | | | |
| | REPS | | | | | | |
| | WEIGHT | | | | | | |
| | REPS | | | | | | |
| | WEIGHT | | | | | | |
| | REPS | | | | | | |
| | WEIGHT | | | | | | |
| | REPS | | | | | | |
| | WEIGHT | | | | | | |
| | REPS | | | | | | |
| | WEIGHT | | | | | | |
| | REPS | | | | | | |

**CARDIO ACTIVITY:**

**NOTES:**

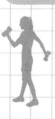

## TIP
Don't have a critical eye? Have someone you trust assess you.

# YOUR TRAINING JOURNAL

**DATE**

| EXERCISE | | SET 1 | SET 2 | SET 3 | SET 4 | SET 5 | SET 6 |
|---|---|---|---|---|---|---|---|
| | WEIGHT | | | | | | |
| | REPS | | | | | | |
| | WEIGHT | | | | | | |
| | REPS | | | | | | |
| | WEIGHT | | | | | | |
| | REPS | | | | | | |
| | WEIGHT | | | | | | |
| | REPS | | | | | | |
| | WEIGHT | | | | | | |
| | REPS | | | | | | |
| | WEIGHT | | | | | | |
| | REPS | | | | | | |
| | WEIGHT | | | | | | |
| | REPS | | | | | | |
| | WEIGHT | | | | | | |
| | REPS | | | | | | |
| | WEIGHT | | | | | | |
| | REPS | | | | | | |
| | WEIGHT | | | | | | |
| | REPS | | | | | | |
| | WEIGHT | | | | | | |
| | REPS | | | | | | |

**CARDIO ACTIVITY:**

**NOTES:**

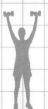

**TIP**

When performing squats, don't let your upper legs go lower than parallel to the floor.

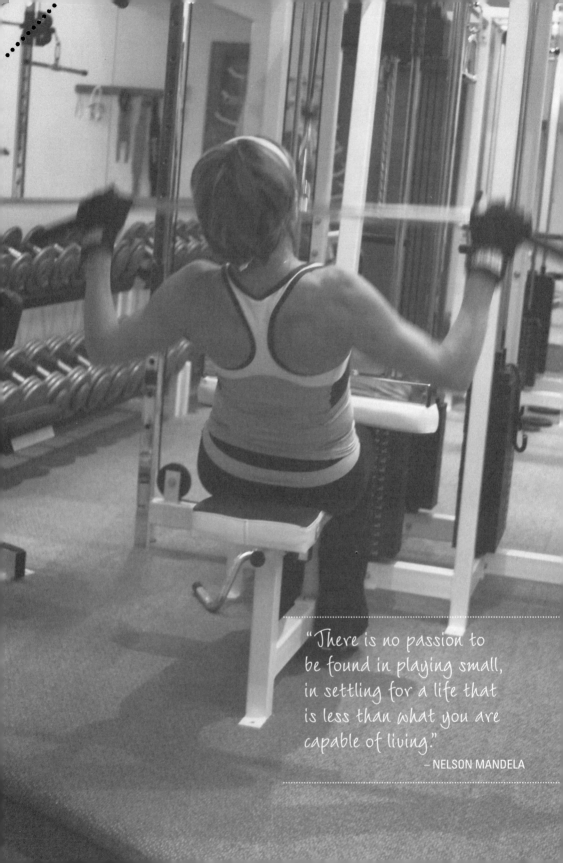

"There is no passion to be found in playing small, in settling for a life that is less than what you are capable of living."

– NELSON MANDELA

# YOUR TRAINING
# JOURNAL

**DATE**

| EXERCISE | | SET 1 | SET 2 | SET 3 | SET 4 | SET 5 | SET 6 |
|---|---|---|---|---|---|---|---|
| | WEIGHT | | | | | | |
| | REPS | | | | | | |
| | WEIGHT | | | | | | |
| | REPS | | | | | | |
| | WEIGHT | | | | | | |
| | REPS | | | | | | |
| | WEIGHT | | | | | | |
| | REPS | | | | | | |
| | WEIGHT | | | | | | |
| | REPS | | | | | | |
| | WEIGHT | | | | | | |
| | REPS | | | | | | |
| | WEIGHT | | | | | | |
| | REPS | | | | | | |
| | WEIGHT | | | | | | |
| | REPS | | | | | | |
| | WEIGHT | | | | | | |
| | REPS | | | | | | |
| | WEIGHT | | | | | | |
| | REPS | | | | | | |
| | WEIGHT | | | | | | |
| | REPS | | | | | | |

**CARDIO ACTIVITY:**

**NOTES:**

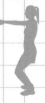

## TIP
Lean back slightly as you pull the bar to the upper chest in the wide-grip pulldown exercise.

# YOUR TRAINING
# JOURNAL

DATE

| EXERCISE | | SET 1 | SET 2 | SET 3 | SET 4 | SET 5 | SET 6 |
|---|---|---|---|---|---|---|---|
| | WEIGHT | | | | | | |
| | REPS | | | | | | |
| | WEIGHT | | | | | | |
| | REPS | | | | | | |
| | WEIGHT | | | | | | |
| | REPS | | | | | | |
| | WEIGHT | | | | | | |
| | REPS | | | | | | |
| | WEIGHT | | | | | | |
| | REPS | | | | | | |
| | WEIGHT | | | | | | |
| | REPS | | | | | | |
| | WEIGHT | | | | | | |
| | REPS | | | | | | |
| | WEIGHT | | | | | | |
| | REPS | | | | | | |
| | WEIGHT | | | | | | |
| | REPS | | | | | | |
| | WEIGHT | | | | | | |
| | REPS | | | | | | |
| | WEIGHT | | | | | | |
| | REPS | | | | | | |

**CARDIO ACTIVITY:**

**NOTES:**

## TIP

*The higher your legs on the leg-press-machine footplate, the more you will improve your butt with the exercise.*

# YOUR TRAINING JOURNAL

**DATE**

| EXERCISE | | SET 1 | SET 2 | SET 3 | SET 4 | SET 5 | SET 6 |
|----------|------|-------|-------|-------|-------|-------|-------|
| | WEIGHT | | | | | | |
| | REPS | | | | | | |
| | WEIGHT | | | | | | |
| | REPS | | | | | | |
| | WEIGHT | | | | | | |
| | REPS | | | | | | |
| | WEIGHT | | | | | | |
| | REPS | | | | | | |
| | WEIGHT | | | | | | |
| | REPS | | | | | | |
| | WEIGHT | | | | | | |
| | REPS | | | | | | |
| | WEIGHT | | | | | | |
| | REPS | | | | | | |
| | WEIGHT | | | | | | |
| | REPS | | | | | | |
| | WEIGHT | | | | | | |
| | REPS | | | | | | |
| | WEIGHT | | | | | | |
| | REPS | | | | | | |
| | WEIGHT | | | | | | |
| | REPS | | | | | | |

**CARDIO ACTIVITY:**

**NOTES:**

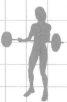

## TIP
Never fail to realize you are what you eat. Consume sugar or fat-loaded junk food and your body will take on the soft, squishy appearance of junk food.

# YOUR TRAINING
# JOURNAL

DATE

| EXERCISE | | SET 1 | SET 2 | SET 3 | SET 4 | SET 5 | SET 6 |
|---|---|---|---|---|---|---|---|
| | WEIGHT | | | | | | |
| | REPS | | | | | | |
| | WEIGHT | | | | | | |
| | REPS | | | | | | |
| | WEIGHT | | | | | | |
| | REPS | | | | | | |
| | WEIGHT | | | | | | |
| | REPS | | | | | | |
| | WEIGHT | | | | | | |
| | REPS | | | | | | |
| | WEIGHT | | | | | | |
| | REPS | | | | | | |
| | WEIGHT | | | | | | |
| | REPS | | | | | | |
| | WEIGHT | | | | | | |
| | REPS | | | | | | |
| | WEIGHT | | | | | | |
| | REPS | | | | | | |
| | WEIGHT | | | | | | |
| | REPS | | | | | | |
| | WEIGHT | | | | | | |
| | REPS | | | | | | |

**CARDIO ACTIVITY:**

**NOTES:**

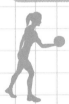

## TIP
Don't get into lengthy conversations between sets.
Keep the training momentum going.

# YOUR TRAINING
# JOURNAL

DATE

| EXERCISE | | SET 1 | SET 2 | SET 3 | SET 4 | SET 5 | SET 6 |
|---|---|---|---|---|---|---|---|
| | WEIGHT | | | | | | |
| | REPS | | | | | | |
| | WEIGHT | | | | | | |
| | REPS | | | | | | |
| | WEIGHT | | | | | | |
| | REPS | | | | | | |
| | WEIGHT | | | | | | |
| | REPS | | | | | | |
| | WEIGHT | | | | | | |
| | REPS | | | | | | |
| | WEIGHT | | | | | | |
| | REPS | | | | | | |
| | WEIGHT | | | | | | |
| | REPS | | | | | | |
| | WEIGHT | | | | | | |
| | REPS | | | | | | |
| | WEIGHT | | | | | | |
| | REPS | | | | | | |
| | WEIGHT | | | | | | |
| | REPS | | | | | | |
| | WEIGHT | | | | | | |
| | REPS | | | | | | |

**CARDIO ACTIVITY:**

**NOTES:**

## TIP
During the dumbell lateral raise, keep your arms slightly bent and turn your hands down as your arms come parallel to the floor — keep little fingers highest.

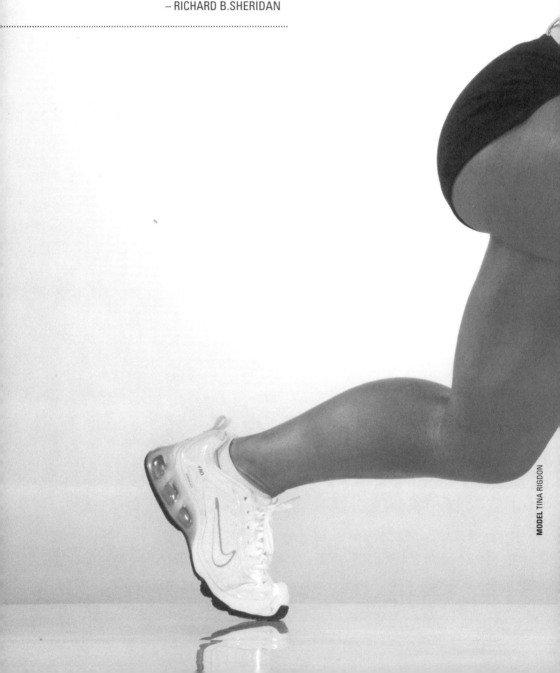

"The surest way not to fail is to determine to succeed."

— RICHARD B.SHERIDAN

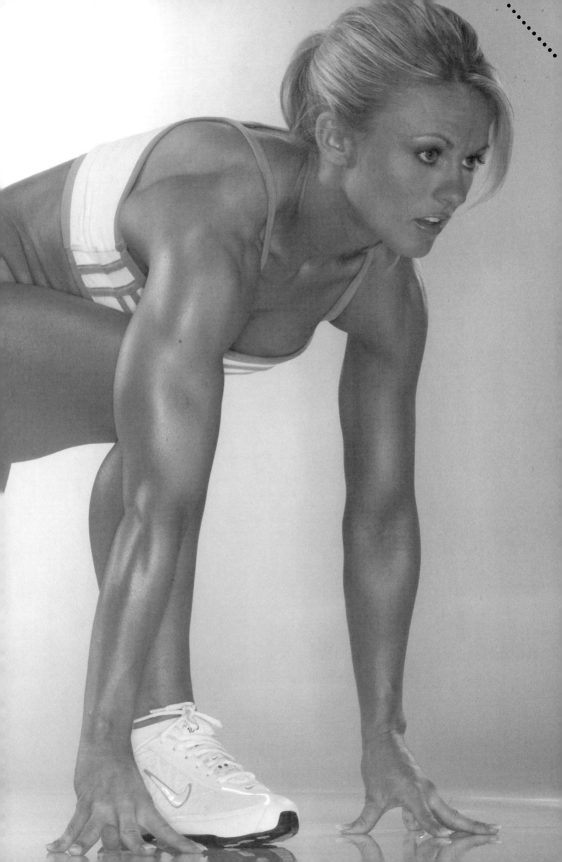

# YOUR TRAINING JOURNAL

DATE

| EXERCISE | | SET 1 | SET 2 | SET 3 | SET 4 | SET 5 | SET 6 |
|---|---|---|---|---|---|---|---|
| | WEIGHT | | | | | | |
| | REPS | | | | | | |
| | WEIGHT | | | | | | |
| | REPS | | | | | | |
| | WEIGHT | | | | | | |
| | REPS | | | | | | |
| | WEIGHT | | | | | | |
| | REPS | | | | | | |
| | WEIGHT | | | | | | |
| | REPS | | | | | | |
| | WEIGHT | | | | | | |
| | REPS | | | | | | |
| | WEIGHT | | | | | | |
| | REPS | | | | | | |
| | WEIGHT | | | | | | |
| | REPS | | | | | | |
| | WEIGHT | | | | | | |
| | REPS | | | | | | |
| | WEIGHT | | | | | | |
| | REPS | | | | | | |
| | WEIGHT | | | | | | |
| | REPS | | | | | | |

**CARDIO ACTIVITY:**

**NOTES:**

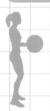

## TIP
When performing cable crossovers, take one step forward to work the outer chest — one step back to work the inner area.

# YOUR TRAINING
# JOURNAL

**DATE**

| EXERCISE | | SET 1 | SET 2 | SET 3 | SET 4 | SET 5 | SET 6 |
|---|---|---|---|---|---|---|---|
| | WEIGHT | | | | | | |
| | REPS | | | | | | |
| | WEIGHT | | | | | | |
| | REPS | | | | | | |
| | WEIGHT | | | | | | |
| | REPS | | | | | | |
| | WEIGHT | | | | | | |
| | REPS | | | | | | |
| | WEIGHT | | | | | | |
| | REPS | | | | | | |
| | WEIGHT | | | | | | |
| | REPS | | | | | | |
| | WEIGHT | | | | | | |
| | REPS | | | | | | |
| | WEIGHT | | | | | | |
| | REPS | | | | | | |
| | WEIGHT | | | | | | |
| | REPS | | | | | | |
| | WEIGHT | | | | | | |
| | REPS | | | | | | |
| | WEIGHT | | | | | | |
| | REPS | | | | | | |

**CARDIO ACTIVITY:**

**NOTES:**

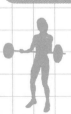

## TIP

Increase your cardio intensity on the treadmill by increasing the incline and by alternating running with walking.

# YOUR TRAINING
# JOURNAL

DATE

| EXERCISE | | SET 1 | SET 2 | SET 3 | SET 4 | SET 5 | SET 6 |
|---|---|---|---|---|---|---|---|
| | WEIGHT | | | | | | |
| | REPS | | | | | | |
| | WEIGHT | | | | | | |
| | REPS | | | | | | |
| | WEIGHT | | | | | | |
| | REPS | | | | | | |
| | WEIGHT | | | | | | |
| | REPS | | | | | | |
| | WEIGHT | | | | | | |
| | REPS | | | | | | |
| | WEIGHT | | | | | | |
| | REPS | | | | | | |
| | WEIGHT | | | | | | |
| | REPS | | | | | | |
| | WEIGHT | | | | | | |
| | REPS | | | | | | |
| | WEIGHT | | | | | | |
| | REPS | | | | | | |
| | WEIGHT | | | | | | |
| | REPS | | | | | | |
| | WEIGHT | | | | | | |
| | REPS | | | | | | |

**CARDIO ACTIVITY:**

**NOTES:**

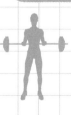

## TIP
When getting back into training after a layoff do just one set of each exercise and build up over a few weeks to regular 3 to 5 sets.

# YOUR TRAINING
# JOURNAL

DATE

| EXERCISE | | SET 1 | SET 2 | SET 3 | SET 4 | SET 5 | SET 6 |
|---|---|---|---|---|---|---|---|
| | WEIGHT | | | | | | |
| | REPS | | | | | | |
| | WEIGHT | | | | | | |
| | REPS | | | | | | |
| | WEIGHT | | | | | | |
| | REPS | | | | | | |
| | WEIGHT | | | | | | |
| | REPS | | | | | | |
| | WEIGHT | | | | | | |
| | REPS | | | | | | |
| | WEIGHT | | | | | | |
| | REPS | | | | | | |
| | WEIGHT | | | | | | |
| | REPS | | | | | | |
| | WEIGHT | | | | | | |
| | REPS | | | | | | |
| | WEIGHT | | | | | | |
| | REPS | | | | | | |
| | WEIGHT | | | | | | |
| | REPS | | | | | | |
| | WEIGHT | | | | | | |
| | REPS | | | | | | |

**CARDIO ACTIVITY:**

**NOTES:**

**TIP**
Train by the clock on occasion. Take no more than
30 seconds of rest between sets.

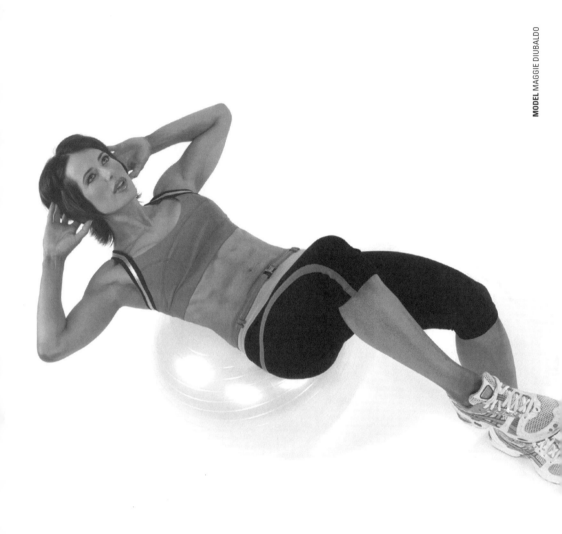

"Determination is the
wake-up call to the
human will."

– ANTHONY ROBBINS

# YOUR TRAINING
# JOURNAL

**DATE**

| EXERCISE | | SET 1 | SET 2 | SET 3 | SET 4 | SET 5 | SET 6 |
|---|---|---|---|---|---|---|---|
| | WEIGHT | | | | | | |
| | REPS | | | | | | |
| | WEIGHT | | | | | | |
| | REPS | | | | | | |
| | WEIGHT | | | | | | |
| | REPS | | | | | | |
| | WEIGHT | | | | | | |
| | REPS | | | | | | |
| | WEIGHT | | | | | | |
| | REPS | | | | | | |
| | WEIGHT | | | | | | |
| | REPS | | | | | | |
| | WEIGHT | | | | | | |
| | REPS | | | | | | |
| | WEIGHT | | | | | | |
| | REPS | | | | | | |
| | WEIGHT | | | | | | |
| | REPS | | | | | | |
| | WEIGHT | | | | | | |
| | REPS | | | | | | |
| | WEIGHT | | | | | | |
| | REPS | | | | | | |

**CARDIO ACTIVITY:**

**NOTES:**

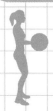

## TIP

Work out your abs by using only lower-abdominal exercises. The upper and middle areas will take care of themselves.

# YOUR TRAINING
# JOURNAL

DATE

| EXERCISE | | SET 1 | SET 2 | SET 3 | SET 4 | SET 5 | SET 6 |
|----------|--------|-------|-------|-------|-------|-------|-------|
| | WEIGHT | | | | | | |
| | REPS | | | | | | |
| | WEIGHT | | | | | | |
| | REPS | | | | | | |
| | WEIGHT | | | | | | |
| | REPS | | | | | | |
| | WEIGHT | | | | | | |
| | REPS | | | | | | |
| | WEIGHT | | | | | | |
| | REPS | | | | | | |
| | WEIGHT | | | | | | |
| | REPS | | | | | | |
| | WEIGHT | | | | | | |
| | REPS | | | | | | |
| | WEIGHT | | | | | | |
| | REPS | | | | | | |
| | WEIGHT | | | | | | |
| | REPS | | | | | | |
| | WEIGHT | | | | | | |
| | REPS | | | | | | |
| | WEIGHT | | | | | | |
| | REPS | | | | | | |

**CARDIO ACTIVITY:**

**NOTES:**

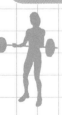

## TIP
Build motivation by checking out your naked body in the mirror and getting upset at what you see.

# YOUR TRAINING JOURNAL

DATE 

| EXERCISE | | SET 1 | SET 2 | SET 3 | SET 4 | SET 5 | SET 6 |
|----------|--------|-------|-------|-------|-------|-------|-------|
| | WEIGHT | | | | | | |
| | REPS | | | | | | |
| | WEIGHT | | | | | | |
| | REPS | | | | | | |
| | WEIGHT | | | | | | |
| | REPS | | | | | | |
| | WEIGHT | | | | | | |
| | REPS | | | | | | |
| | WEIGHT | | | | | | |
| | REPS | | | | | | |
| | WEIGHT | | | | | | |
| | REPS | | | | | | |
| | WEIGHT | | | | | | |
| | REPS | | | | | | |
| | WEIGHT | | | | | | |
| | REPS | | | | | | |
| | WEIGHT | | | | | | |
| | REPS | | | | | | |
| | WEIGHT | | | | | | |
| | REPS | | | | | | |
| | WEIGHT | | | | | | |
| | REPS | | | | | | |

**CARDIO ACTIVITY:**

**NOTES:**

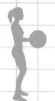

**TIP**
Always take a towel to the gym. The MRSA bacteria are with us.

# YOUR TRAINING JOURNAL

DATE

| EXERCISE | | SET 1 | SET 2 | SET 3 | SET 4 | SET 5 | SET 6 |
|---|---|---|---|---|---|---|---|
| | WEIGHT | | | | | | |
| | REPS | | | | | | |
| | WEIGHT | | | | | | |
| | REPS | | | | | | |
| | WEIGHT | | | | | | |
| | REPS | | | | | | |
| | WEIGHT | | | | | | |
| | REPS | | | | | | |
| | WEIGHT | | | | | | |
| | REPS | | | | | | |
| | WEIGHT | | | | | | |
| | REPS | | | | | | |
| | WEIGHT | | | | | | |
| | REPS | | | | | | |
| | WEIGHT | | | | | | |
| | REPS | | | | | | |
| | WEIGHT | | | | | | |
| | REPS | | | | | | |
| | WEIGHT | | | | | | |
| | REPS | | | | | | |
| | WEIGHT | | | | | | |
| | REPS | | | | | | |

**CARDIO ACTIVITY:**

**NOTES:**

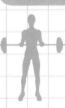

## TIP
Every exercise should start with a warm-up set of 20 repetitions with a lighter weight.

# YOUR TRAINING JOURNAL

DATE

| EXERCISE | | SET 1 | SET 2 | SET 3 | SET 4 | SET 5 | SET 6 |
|---|---|---|---|---|---|---|---|
| | WEIGHT | | | | | | |
| | REPS | | | | | | |
| | WEIGHT | | | | | | |
| | REPS | | | | | | |
| | WEIGHT | | | | | | |
| | REPS | | | | | | |
| | WEIGHT | | | | | | |
| | REPS | | | | | | |
| | WEIGHT | | | | | | |
| | REPS | | | | | | |
| | WEIGHT | | | | | | |
| | REPS | | | | | | |
| | WEIGHT | | | | | | |
| | REPS | | | | | | |
| | WEIGHT | | | | | | |
| | REPS | | | | | | |
| | WEIGHT | | | | | | |
| | REPS | | | | | | |
| | WEIGHT | | | | | | |
| | REPS | | | | | | |
| | WEIGHT | | | | | | |
| | REPS | | | | | | |

**CARDIO ACTIVITY:**

**NOTES:**

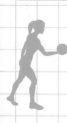

## TIP
Eating out? Be polite but firm. Request no sauce, no sour cream and no bacon bits. Ask for steamed veggies, a baked or grilled entrée and no butter! Have fresh fruit or berries for dessert.

# YOUR TRAINING JOURNAL

DATE

| EXERCISE | | SET 1 | SET 2 | SET 3 | SET 4 | SET 5 | SET 6 |
|---|---|---|---|---|---|---|---|
| | WEIGHT | | | | | | |
| | REPS | | | | | | |
| | WEIGHT | | | | | | |
| | REPS | | | | | | |
| | WEIGHT | | | | | | |
| | REPS | | | | | | |
| | WEIGHT | | | | | | |
| | REPS | | | | | | |
| | WEIGHT | | | | | | |
| | REPS | | | | | | |
| | WEIGHT | | | | | | |
| | REPS | | | | | | |
| | WEIGHT | | | | | | |
| | REPS | | | | | | |
| | WEIGHT | | | | | | |
| | REPS | | | | | | |
| | WEIGHT | | | | | | |
| | REPS | | | | | | |
| | WEIGHT | | | | | | |
| | REPS | | | | | | |
| | WEIGHT | | | | | | |
| | REPS | | | | | | |

**CARDIO ACTIVITY:**

**NOTES:**

**TIP**

Avoid anabolic drugs and growth hormone. The end result is a huge health problem.

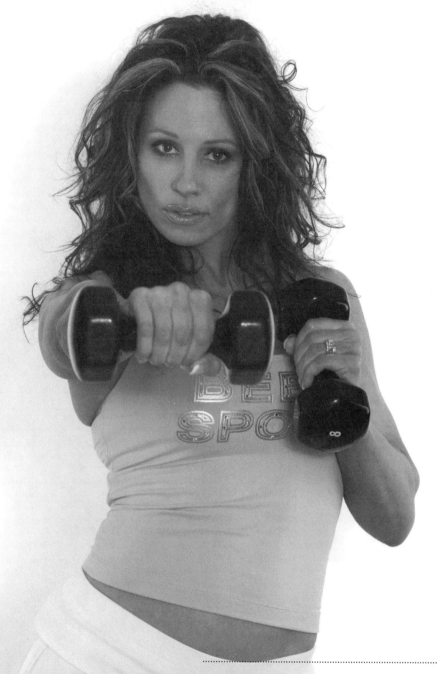

"The best way out is
always through."

– ROBERT FROST

# YOUR TRAINING
# JOURNAL

**DATE**

| EXERCISE | | SET 1 | SET 2 | SET 3 | SET 4 | SET 5 | SET 6 |
|---|---|---|---|---|---|---|---|
| | WEIGHT | | | | | | |
| | REPS | | | | | | |
| | WEIGHT | | | | | | |
| | REPS | | | | | | |
| | WEIGHT | | | | | | |
| | REPS | | | | | | |
| | WEIGHT | | | | | | |
| | REPS | | | | | | |
| | WEIGHT | | | | | | |
| | REPS | | | | | | |
| | WEIGHT | | | | | | |
| | REPS | | | | | | |
| | WEIGHT | | | | | | |
| | REPS | | | | | | |
| | WEIGHT | | | | | | |
| | REPS | | | | | | |
| | WEIGHT | | | | | | |
| | REPS | | | | | | |
| | WEIGHT | | | | | | |
| | REPS | | | | | | |
| | WEIGHT | | | | | | |
| | REPS | | | | | | |

**CARDIO ACTIVITY:**

**NOTES:**

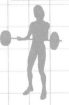

## TIP
Carry yourself with dignity both in and out of the gym. Keep your posture strong.

# YOUR TRAINING JOURNAL

DATE

| EXERCISE | | SET 1 | SET 2 | SET 3 | SET 4 | SET 5 | SET 6 |
|----------|---|-------|-------|-------|-------|-------|-------|
| | WEIGHT | | | | | | |
| | REPS | | | | | | |
| | WEIGHT | | | | | | |
| | REPS | | | | | | |
| | WEIGHT | | | | | | |
| | REPS | | | | | | |
| | WEIGHT | | | | | | |
| | REPS | | | | | | |
| | WEIGHT | | | | | | |
| | REPS | | | | | | |
| | WEIGHT | | | | | | |
| | REPS | | | | | | |
| | WEIGHT | | | | | | |
| | REPS | | | | | | |
| | WEIGHT | | | | | | |
| | REPS | | | | | | |
| | WEIGHT | | | | | | |
| | REPS | | | | | | |
| | WEIGHT | | | | | | |
| | REPS | | | | | | |
| | WEIGHT | | | | | | |
| | REPS | | | | | | |

**CARDIO ACTIVITY:**

**NOTES:**

## TIP
Use alcohol wipes to clean off the bench you have just employed, even if you used a towel.

# YOUR TRAINING
# JOURNAL

**DATE**

| EXERCISE | | SET 1 | SET 2 | SET 3 | SET 4 | SET 5 | SET 6 |
|---|---|---|---|---|---|---|---|
| | WEIGHT | | | | | | |
| | REPS | | | | | | |
| | WEIGHT | | | | | | |
| | REPS | | | | | | |
| | WEIGHT | | | | | | |
| | REPS | | | | | | |
| | WEIGHT | | | | | | |
| | REPS | | | | | | |
| | WEIGHT | | | | | | |
| | REPS | | | | | | |
| | WEIGHT | | | | | | |
| | REPS | | | | | | |
| | WEIGHT | | | | | | |
| | REPS | | | | | | |
| | WEIGHT | | | | | | |
| | REPS | | | | | | |
| | WEIGHT | | | | | | |
| | REPS | | | | | | |
| | WEIGHT | | | | | | |
| | REPS | | | | | | |
| | WEIGHT | | | | | | |
| | REPS | | | | | | |

**CARDIO ACTIVITY:**

**NOTES:**

## TIP
Keep your workout brief and focused. Don't waste time.

# YOUR TRAINING
# JOURNAL

**DATE**

| EXERCISE | | SET 1 | SET 2 | SET 3 | SET 4 | SET 5 | SET 6 |
|---|---|---|---|---|---|---|---|
| | WEIGHT | | | | | | |
| | REPS | | | | | | |
| | WEIGHT | | | | | | |
| | REPS | | | | | | |
| | WEIGHT | | | | | | |
| | REPS | | | | | | |
| | WEIGHT | | | | | | |
| | REPS | | | | | | |
| | WEIGHT | | | | | | |
| | REPS | | | | | | |
| | WEIGHT | | | | | | |
| | REPS | | | | | | |
| | WEIGHT | | | | | | |
| | REPS | | | | | | |
| | WEIGHT | | | | | | |
| | REPS | | | | | | |
| | WEIGHT | | | | | | |
| | REPS | | | | | | |
| | WEIGHT | | | | | | |
| | REPS | | | | | | |
| | WEIGHT | | | | | | |
| | REPS | | | | | | |

**CARDIO ACTIVITY:**

**NOTES:**

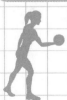

## TIP
Plan your eating in advance. To save time, cook planned extras.

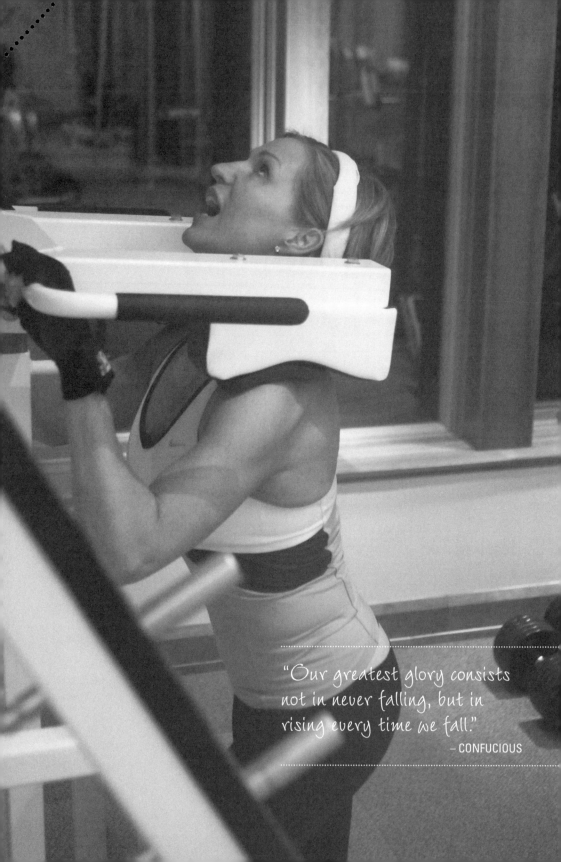

"Our greatest glory consists not in never falling, but in rising every time we fall."

– CONFUCIOUS

# YOUR TRAINING JOURNAL

DATE

| EXERCISE | | SET 1 | SET 2 | SET 3 | SET 4 | SET 5 | SET 6 |
|---|---|---|---|---|---|---|---|
| | WEIGHT | | | | | | |
| | REPS | | | | | | |
| | WEIGHT | | | | | | |
| | REPS | | | | | | |
| | WEIGHT | | | | | | |
| | REPS | | | | | | |
| | WEIGHT | | | | | | |
| | REPS | | | | | | |
| | WEIGHT | | | | | | |
| | REPS | | | | | | |
| | WEIGHT | | | | | | |
| | REPS | | | | | | |
| | WEIGHT | | | | | | |
| | REPS | | | | | | |
| | WEIGHT | | | | | | |
| | REPS | | | | | | |
| | WEIGHT | | | | | | |
| | REPS | | | | | | |
| | WEIGHT | | | | | | |
| | REPS | | | | | | |
| | WEIGHT | | | | | | |
| | REPS | | | | | | |

**CARDIO ACTIVITY:**

**NOTES:**

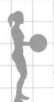

## TIP
After a layoff don't try and resume training where you left off. Using the same heavy weights is not an option.

# YOUR TRAINING
# JOURNAL

DATE

| EXERCISE | | SET 1 | SET 2 | SET 3 | SET 4 | SET 5 | SET 6 |
|---|---|---|---|---|---|---|---|
| | WEIGHT | | | | | | |
| | REPS | | | | | | |
| | WEIGHT | | | | | | |
| | REPS | | | | | | |
| | WEIGHT | | | | | | |
| | REPS | | | | | | |
| | WEIGHT | | | | | | |
| | REPS | | | | | | |
| | WEIGHT | | | | | | |
| | REPS | | | | | | |
| | WEIGHT | | | | | | |
| | REPS | | | | | | |
| | WEIGHT | | | | | | |
| | REPS | | | | | | |
| | WEIGHT | | | | | | |
| | REPS | | | | | | |
| | WEIGHT | | | | | | |
| | REPS | | | | | | |
| | WEIGHT | | | | | | |
| | REPS | | | | | | |
| | WEIGHT | | | | | | |
| | REPS | | | | | | |

**CARDIO ACTIVITY:**

**NOTES:**

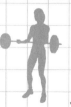

## TIP

Try the Arnold press for delts. Start with the dumbells at the shoulders, then as you press them upwards rotate your hands until the palms are facing out.

# YOUR TRAINING JOURNAL

**DATE**

| EXERCISE | | SET 1 | SET 2 | SET 3 | SET 4 | SET 5 | SET 6 |
|---|---|---|---|---|---|---|---|
| | WEIGHT | | | | | | |
| | REPS | | | | | | |
| | WEIGHT | | | | | | |
| | REPS | | | | | | |
| | WEIGHT | | | | | | |
| | REPS | | | | | | |
| | WEIGHT | | | | | | |
| | REPS | | | | | | |
| | WEIGHT | | | | | | |
| | REPS | | | | | | |
| | WEIGHT | | | | | | |
| | REPS | | | | | | |
| | WEIGHT | | | | | | |
| | REPS | | | | | | |
| | WEIGHT | | | | | | |
| | REPS | | | | | | |
| | WEIGHT | | | | | | |
| | REPS | | | | | | |
| | WEIGHT | | | | | | |
| | REPS | | | | | | |
| | WEIGHT | | | | | | |
| | REPS | | | | | | |

**CARDIO ACTIVITY:**

**NOTES:**

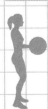

**TIP**

To make your barbell curls super strict, lean back against an upright post or wall.

# YOUR TRAINING JOURNAL

**DATE**

| EXERCISE | | SET 1 | SET 2 | SET 3 | SET 4 | SET 5 | SET 6 |
|---|---|---|---|---|---|---|---|
| | WEIGHT | | | | | | |
| | REPS | | | | | | |
| | WEIGHT | | | | | | |
| | REPS | | | | | | |
| | WEIGHT | | | | | | |
| | REPS | | | | | | |
| | WEIGHT | | | | | | |
| | REPS | | | | | | |
| | WEIGHT | | | | | | |
| | REPS | | | | | | |
| | WEIGHT | | | | | | |
| | REPS | | | | | | |
| | WEIGHT | | | | | | |
| | REPS | | | | | | |
| | WEIGHT | | | | | | |
| | REPS | | | | | | |
| | WEIGHT | | | | | | |
| | REPS | | | | | | |
| | WEIGHT | | | | | | |
| | REPS | | | | | | |
| | WEIGHT | | | | | | |
| | REPS | | | | | | |

**CARDIO ACTIVITY:**

**NOTES:**

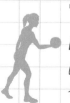

## TIP

When performing triceps pushdowns, keep the elbows wide to hit the outer triceps head. Keep elbows tight to the body for triceps mass.

# YOUR TRAINING JOURNAL

DATE

| EXERCISE | | SET 1 | SET 2 | SET 3 | SET 4 | SET 5 | SET 6 |
|---|---|---|---|---|---|---|---|
| | WEIGHT | | | | | | |
| | REPS | | | | | | |
| | WEIGHT | | | | | | |
| | REPS | | | | | | |
| | WEIGHT | | | | | | |
| | REPS | | | | | | |
| | WEIGHT | | | | | | |
| | REPS | | | | | | |
| | WEIGHT | | | | | | |
| | REPS | | | | | | |
| | WEIGHT | | | | | | |
| | REPS | | | | | | |
| | WEIGHT | | | | | | |
| | REPS | | | | | | |
| | WEIGHT | | | | | | |
| | REPS | | | | | | |
| | WEIGHT | | | | | | |
| | REPS | | | | | | |
| | WEIGHT | | | | | | |
| | REPS | | | | | | |
| | WEIGHT | | | | | | |
| | REPS | | | | | | |

**CARDIO ACTIVITY:**

**NOTES:**

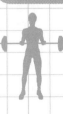

## TIP
Breathe deeply when exercising. Gulp air through the mouth, especially in heavy exercises like squats or bench press.

# YOUR TRAINING
# JOURNAL

DATE

| EXERCISE | | SET 1 | SET 2 | SET 3 | SET 4 | SET 5 | SET 6 |
|---|---|---|---|---|---|---|---|
| | WEIGHT | | | | | | |
| | REPS | | | | | | |
| | WEIGHT | | | | | | |
| | REPS | | | | | | |
| | WEIGHT | | | | | | |
| | REPS | | | | | | |
| | WEIGHT | | | | | | |
| | REPS | | | | | | |
| | WEIGHT | | | | | | |
| | REPS | | | | | | |
| | WEIGHT | | | | | | |
| | REPS | | | | | | |
| | WEIGHT | | | | | | |
| | REPS | | | | | | |
| | WEIGHT | | | | | | |
| | REPS | | | | | | |
| | WEIGHT | | | | | | |
| | REPS | | | | | | |
| | WEIGHT | | | | | | |
| | REPS | | | | | | |
| | WEIGHT | | | | | | |
| | REPS | | | | | | |

**CARDIO ACTIVITY:**

**NOTES:**

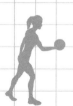

## TIP
Want rounder glutes? Go for the low-cable bench kickbacks.

# YOUR TRAINING JOURNAL

DATE

| EXERCISE | | SET 1 | SET 2 | SET 3 | SET 4 | SET 5 | SET 6 |
|---|---|---|---|---|---|---|---|
| | WEIGHT | | | | | | |
| | REPS | | | | | | |
| | WEIGHT | | | | | | |
| | REPS | | | | | | |
| | WEIGHT | | | | | | |
| | REPS | | | | | | |
| | WEIGHT | | | | | | |
| | REPS | | | | | | |
| | WEIGHT | | | | | | |
| | REPS | | | | | | |
| | WEIGHT | | | | | | |
| | REPS | | | | | | |
| | WEIGHT | | | | | | |
| | REPS | | | | | | |
| | WEIGHT | | | | | | |
| | REPS | | | | | | |
| | WEIGHT | | | | | | |
| | REPS | | | | | | |
| | WEIGHT | | | | | | |
| | REPS | | | | | | |
| | WEIGHT | | | | | | |
| | REPS | | | | | | |

**CARDIO ACTIVITY:**

**NOTES:**

## TIP
Don't hog the equipment at a public gym. Get up off the bench you have been using so others can take their turn.

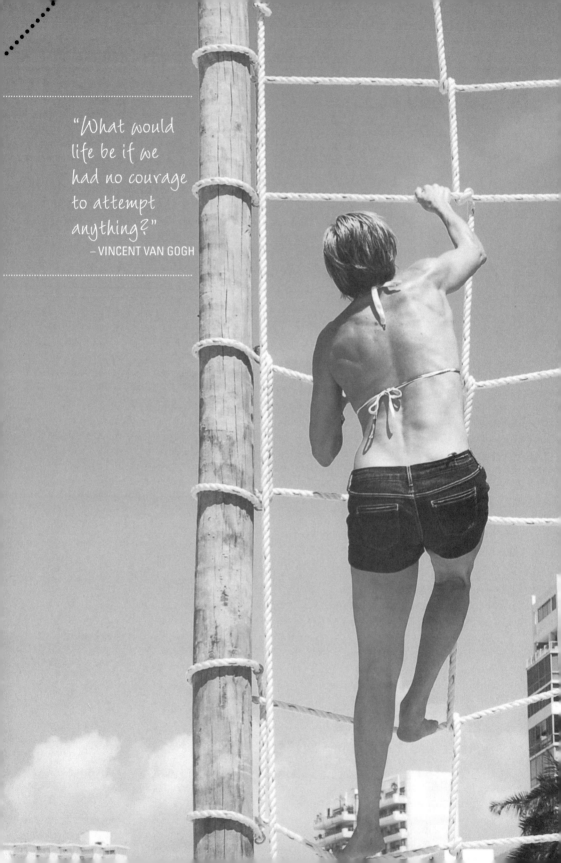

"What would life be if we had no courage to attempt anything?"
– VINCENT VAN GOGH

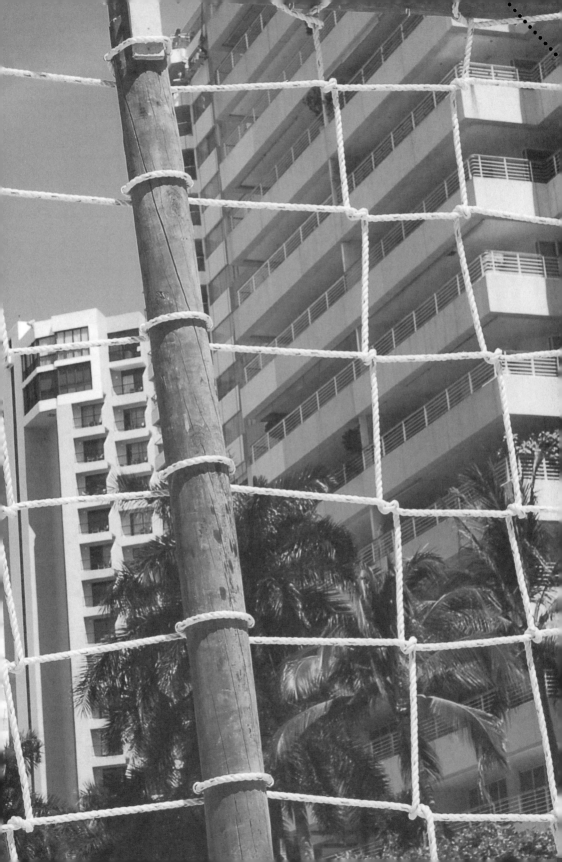

# YOUR TRAINING
# JOURNAL

**DATE**

| EXERCISE | | SET 1 | SET 2 | SET 3 | SET 4 | SET 5 | SET 6 |
|---|---|---|---|---|---|---|---|
| | WEIGHT | | | | | | |
| | REPS | | | | | | |
| | WEIGHT | | | | | | |
| | REPS | | | | | | |
| | WEIGHT | | | | | | |
| | REPS | | | | | | |
| | WEIGHT | | | | | | |
| | REPS | | | | | | |
| | WEIGHT | | | | | | |
| | REPS | | | | | | |
| | WEIGHT | | | | | | |
| | REPS | | | | | | |
| | WEIGHT | | | | | | |
| | REPS | | | | | | |
| | WEIGHT | | | | | | |
| | REPS | | | | | | |
| | WEIGHT | | | | | | |
| | REPS | | | | | | |
| | WEIGHT | | | | | | |
| | REPS | | | | | | |
| | WEIGHT | | | | | | |
| | REPS | | | | | | |

**CARDIO ACTIVITY:**

**NOTES:**

## TIP
Don't eat three big meals a day. Eat smaller meals, each containing a complex carb and lean protein.

# YOUR TRAINING JOURNAL

DATE

| EXERCISE | | SET 1 | SET 2 | SET 3 | SET 4 | SET 5 | SET 6 |
|---|---|---|---|---|---|---|---|
| | WEIGHT | | | | | | |
| | REPS | | | | | | |
| | WEIGHT | | | | | | |
| | REPS | | | | | | |
| | WEIGHT | | | | | | |
| | REPS | | | | | | |
| | WEIGHT | | | | | | |
| | REPS | | | | | | |
| | WEIGHT | | | | | | |
| | REPS | | | | | | |
| | WEIGHT | | | | | | |
| | REPS | | | | | | |
| | WEIGHT | | | | | | |
| | REPS | | | | | | |
| | WEIGHT | | | | | | |
| | REPS | | | | | | |
| | WEIGHT | | | | | | |
| | REPS | | | | | | |
| | WEIGHT | | | | | | |
| | REPS | | | | | | |
| | WEIGHT | | | | | | |
| | REPS | | | | | | |

**CARDIO ACTIVITY:**

**NOTES:**

## TIP

Take a multivitamin supplement and whey protein powder to keep your nutrition and cell repair on track.

# YOUR TRAINING
# JOURNAL

DATE

| EXERCISE | | SET 1 | SET 2 | SET 3 | SET 4 | SET 5 | SET 6 |
|---|---|---|---|---|---|---|---|
| | WEIGHT | | | | | | |
| | REPS | | | | | | |
| | WEIGHT | | | | | | |
| | REPS | | | | | | |
| | WEIGHT | | | | | | |
| | REPS | | | | | | |
| | WEIGHT | | | | | | |
| | REPS | | | | | | |
| | WEIGHT | | | | | | |
| | REPS | | | | | | |
| | WEIGHT | | | | | | |
| | REPS | | | | | | |
| | WEIGHT | | | | | | |
| | REPS | | | | | | |
| | WEIGHT | | | | | | |
| | REPS | | | | | | |
| | WEIGHT | | | | | | |
| | REPS | | | | | | |
| | WEIGHT | | | | | | |
| | REPS | | | | | | |
| | WEIGHT | | | | | | |
| | REPS | | | | | | |

**CARDIO ACTIVITY:**

**NOTES:**

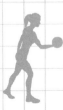

## TIP
Don't bulk up with heavy eating and heavy weights.
Even muscular bulk can be hard to get rid of when bikini
weather comes around.

"If you do not hope,
you will not find what is
beyond your hopes."
– ST. CLEMENT OF ALEXANDRIA

# YOUR TRAINING
# JOURNAL

DATE

| EXERCISE | | SET 1 | SET 2 | SET 3 | SET 4 | SET 5 | SET 6 |
|----------|---|-------|-------|-------|-------|-------|-------|
| | WEIGHT | | | | | | |
| | REPS | | | | | | |
| | WEIGHT | | | | | | |
| | REPS | | | | | | |
| | WEIGHT | | | | | | |
| | REPS | | | | | | |
| | WEIGHT | | | | | | |
| | REPS | | | | | | |
| | WEIGHT | | | | | | |
| | REPS | | | | | | |
| | WEIGHT | | | | | | |
| | REPS | | | | | | |
| | WEIGHT | | | | | | |
| | REPS | | | | | | |
| | WEIGHT | | | | | | |
| | REPS | | | | | | |
| | WEIGHT | | | | | | |
| | REPS | | | | | | |
| | WEIGHT | | | | | | |
| | REPS | | | | | | |
| | WEIGHT | | | | | | |
| | REPS | | | | | | |

**CARDIO ACTIVITY:**

**NOTES:**

## TIP
When performing Smith-machine squats, stand one step back from the machine to work your glutes and one step forward to work your lower quads.

# YOUR TRAINING
# JOURNAL

DATE

| EXERCISE | | SET 1 | SET 2 | SET 3 | SET 4 | SET 5 | SET 6 |
|---|---|---|---|---|---|---|---|
| | WEIGHT | | | | | | |
| | REPS | | | | | | |
| | WEIGHT | | | | | | |
| | REPS | | | | | | |
| | WEIGHT | | | | | | |
| | REPS | | | | | | |
| | WEIGHT | | | | | | |
| | REPS | | | | | | |
| | WEIGHT | | | | | | |
| | REPS | | | | | | |
| | WEIGHT | | | | | | |
| | REPS | | | | | | |
| | WEIGHT | | | | | | |
| | REPS | | | | | | |
| | WEIGHT | | | | | | |
| | REPS | | | | | | |
| | WEIGHT | | | | | | |
| | REPS | | | | | | |
| | WEIGHT | | | | | | |
| | REPS | | | | | | |
| | WEIGHT | | | | | | |
| | REPS | | | | | | |

**CARDIO ACTIVITY:**

**NOTES:**

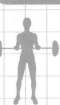

## TIP
Don't practice regular situps. Crunches are a more direct and effective ab exercise.

# YOUR TRAINING
# JOURNAL

DATE

| EXERCISE | | SET 1 | SET 2 | SET 3 | SET 4 | SET 5 | SET 6 |
|---|---|---|---|---|---|---|---|
| | WEIGHT | | | | | | |
| | REPS | | | | | | |
| | WEIGHT | | | | | | |
| | REPS | | | | | | |
| | WEIGHT | | | | | | |
| | REPS | | | | | | |
| | WEIGHT | | | | | | |
| | REPS | | | | | | |
| | WEIGHT | | | | | | |
| | REPS | | | | | | |
| | WEIGHT | | | | | | |
| | REPS | | | | | | |
| | WEIGHT | | | | | | |
| | REPS | | | | | | |
| | WEIGHT | | | | | | |
| | REPS | | | | | | |
| | WEIGHT | | | | | | |
| | REPS | | | | | | |
| | WEIGHT | | | | | | |
| | REPS | | | | | | |
| | WEIGHT | | | | | | |
| | REPS | | | | | | |

**CARDIO ACTIVITY:**

**NOTES:**

## TIP
Always wear supportive footwear in the gym.

# YOUR TRAINING JOURNAL

**DATE**

| EXERCISE | | SET 1 | SET 2 | SET 3 | SET 4 | SET 5 | SET 6 |
|---|---|---|---|---|---|---|---|
| | WEIGHT | | | | | | |
| | REPS | | | | | | |
| | WEIGHT | | | | | | |
| | REPS | | | | | | |
| | WEIGHT | | | | | | |
| | REPS | | | | | | |
| | WEIGHT | | | | | | |
| | REPS | | | | | | |
| | WEIGHT | | | | | | |
| | REPS | | | | | | |
| | WEIGHT | | | | | | |
| | REPS | | | | | | |
| | WEIGHT | | | | | | |
| | REPS | | | | | | |
| | WEIGHT | | | | | | |
| | REPS | | | | | | |
| | WEIGHT | | | | | | |
| | REPS | | | | | | |
| | WEIGHT | | | | | | |
| | REPS | | | | | | |
| | WEIGHT | | | | | | |
| | REPS | | | | | | |

**CARDIO ACTIVITY:**

**NOTES:**

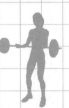

## TIP
Sneakers worn every day should be replaced every six months.

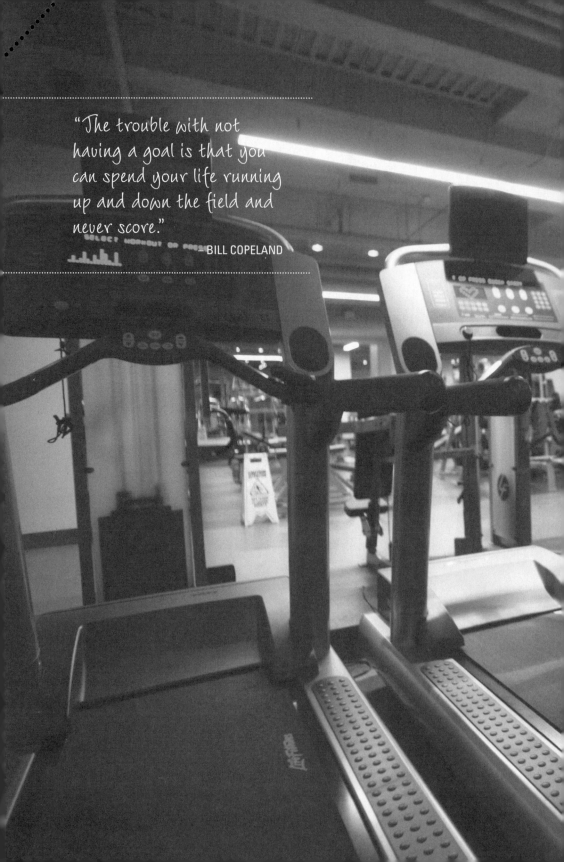

"The trouble with not
having a goal is that you
can spend your life running
up and down the field and
never score."

BILL COPELAND

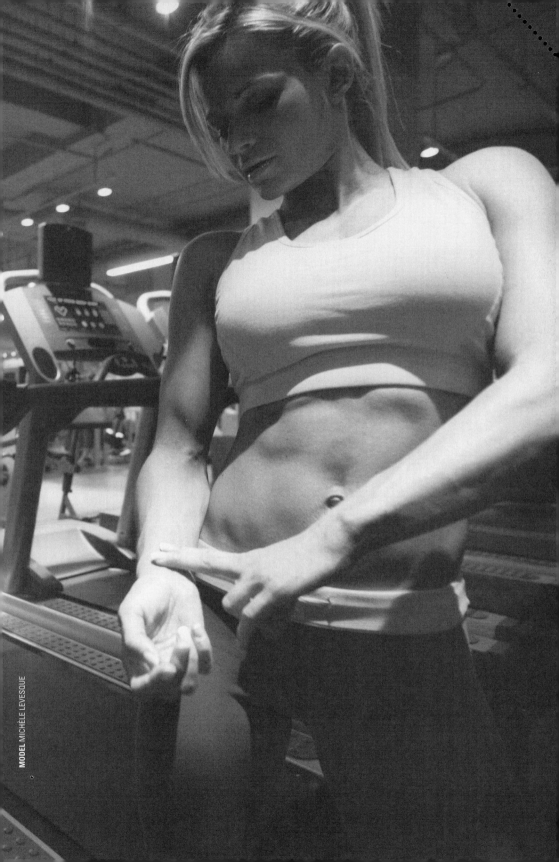

# YOUR TRAINING JOURNAL

DATE

| EXERCISE | | SET 1 | SET 2 | SET 3 | SET 4 | SET 5 | SET 6 |
|---|---|---|---|---|---|---|---|
| | WEIGHT | | | | | | |
| | REPS | | | | | | |
| | WEIGHT | | | | | | |
| | REPS | | | | | | |
| | WEIGHT | | | | | | |
| | REPS | | | | | | |
| | WEIGHT | | | | | | |
| | REPS | | | | | | |
| | WEIGHT | | | | | | |
| | REPS | | | | | | |
| | WEIGHT | | | | | | |
| | REPS | | | | | | |
| | WEIGHT | | | | | | |
| | REPS | | | | | | |
| | WEIGHT | | | | | | |
| | REPS | | | | | | |
| | WEIGHT | | | | | | |
| | REPS | | | | | | |
| | WEIGHT | | | | | | |
| | REPS | | | | | | |
| | WEIGHT | | | | | | |
| | REPS | | | | | | |

**CARDIO ACTIVITY:**

**NOTES:**

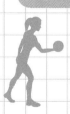

## TIP
Good pain. Bad pain. Learn to understand the difference. If you feel a twinge or tear in your muscles, stop that exercise immediately.

# YOUR TRAINING JOURNAL

**DATE**

| EXERCISE | | SET 1 | SET 2 | SET 3 | SET 4 | SET 5 | SET 6 |
|---|---|---|---|---|---|---|---|
| | WEIGHT | | | | | | |
| | REPS | | | | | | |
| | WEIGHT | | | | | | |
| | REPS | | | | | | |
| | WEIGHT | | | | | | |
| | REPS | | | | | | |
| | WEIGHT | | | | | | |
| | REPS | | | | | | |
| | WEIGHT | | | | | | |
| | REPS | | | | | | |
| | WEIGHT | | | | | | |
| | REPS | | | | | | |
| | WEIGHT | | | | | | |
| | REPS | | | | | | |
| | WEIGHT | | | | | | |
| | REPS | | | | | | |
| | WEIGHT | | | | | | |
| | REPS | | | | | | |
| | WEIGHT | | | | | | |
| | REPS | | | | | | |
| | WEIGHT | | | | | | |
| | REPS | | | | | | |

**CARDIO ACTIVITY:**

**NOTES:**

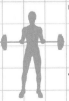

## TIP

Constant evaluation is vital. Learn to really see yourself. Ask a trusted friend for an honest opinion if in doubt.

# YOUR TRAINING JOURNAL

DATE

| EXERCISE | | SET 1 | SET 2 | SET 3 | SET 4 | SET 5 | SET 6 |
|---|---|---|---|---|---|---|---|
| | WEIGHT | | | | | | |
| | REPS | | | | | | |
| | WEIGHT | | | | | | |
| | REPS | | | | | | |
| | WEIGHT | | | | | | |
| | REPS | | | | | | |
| | WEIGHT | | | | | | |
| | REPS | | | | | | |
| | WEIGHT | | | | | | |
| | REPS | | | | | | |
| | WEIGHT | | | | | | |
| | REPS | | | | | | |
| | WEIGHT | | | | | | |
| | REPS | | | | | | |
| | WEIGHT | | | | | | |
| | REPS | | | | | | |
| | WEIGHT | | | | | | |
| | REPS | | | | | | |
| | WEIGHT | | | | | | |
| | REPS | | | | | | |
| | WEIGHT | | | | | | |
| | REPS | | | | | | |

**CARDIO ACTIVITY:**

**NOTES:**

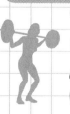

## TIP

If weights are not available try pushups, squats, crunches and other exercises using body weight. A little exercise is better than none.

# YOUR TRAINING JOURNAL

DATE

| EXERCISE | | SET 1 | SET 2 | SET 3 | SET 4 | SET 5 | SET 6 |
|---|---|---|---|---|---|---|---|
| | WEIGHT | | | | | | |
| | REPS | | | | | | |
| | WEIGHT | | | | | | |
| | REPS | | | | | | |
| | WEIGHT | | | | | | |
| | REPS | | | | | | |
| | WEIGHT | | | | | | |
| | REPS | | | | | | |
| | WEIGHT | | | | | | |
| | REPS | | | | | | |
| | WEIGHT | | | | | | |
| | REPS | | | | | | |
| | WEIGHT | | | | | | |
| | REPS | | | | | | |
| | WEIGHT | | | | | | |
| | REPS | | | | | | |
| | WEIGHT | | | | | | |
| | REPS | | | | | | |
| | WEIGHT | | | | | | |
| | REPS | | | | | | |
| | WEIGHT | | | | | | |
| | REPS | | | | | | |

**CARDIO ACTIVITY:**

**NOTES:**

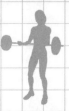

## TIP

If you train at home and want serious results, use squat racks and an adjustable flat/incline bench as minimum apparatus requirements.

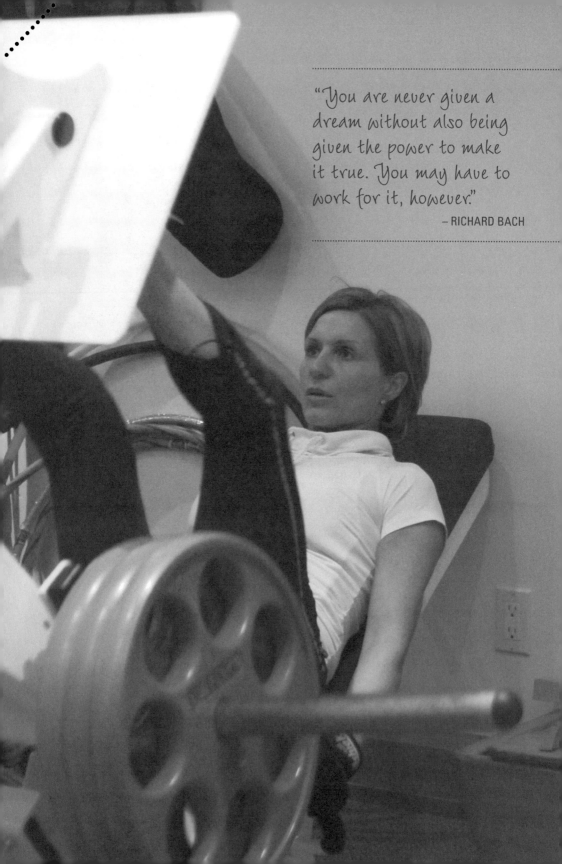

"You are never given a dream without also being given the power to make it true. You may have to work for it, however."

— RICHARD BACH

# YOUR TRAINING JOURNAL

**DATE**

| EXERCISE | | SET 1 | SET 2 | SET 3 | SET 4 | SET 5 | SET 6 |
|---|---|---|---|---|---|---|---|
| | WEIGHT | | | | | | |
| | REPS | | | | | | |
| | WEIGHT | | | | | | |
| | REPS | | | | | | |
| | WEIGHT | | | | | | |
| | REPS | | | | | | |
| | WEIGHT | | | | | | |
| | REPS | | | | | | |
| | WEIGHT | | | | | | |
| | REPS | | | | | | |
| | WEIGHT | | | | | | |
| | REPS | | | | | | |
| | WEIGHT | | | | | | |
| | REPS | | | | | | |
| | WEIGHT | | | | | | |
| | REPS | | | | | | |
| | WEIGHT | | | | | | |
| | REPS | | | | | | |
| | WEIGHT | | | | | | |
| | REPS | | | | | | |
| | WEIGHT | | | | | | |
| | REPS | | | | | | |

**CARDIO ACTIVITY:**

**NOTES:**

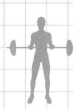

**TIP**

Constantly seek knowledge by subscribing to at least one of the following: Oxygen, Muscle & Fitness Hers, Maximum Fitness or Reps!

# YOUR TRAINING
# JOURNAL

**DATE**

| EXERCISE | | SET 1 | SET 2 | SET 3 | SET 4 | SET 5 | SET 6 |
|---|---|---|---|---|---|---|---|
| | WEIGHT | | | | | | |
| | REPS | | | | | | |
| | WEIGHT | | | | | | |
| | REPS | | | | | | |
| | WEIGHT | | | | | | |
| | REPS | | | | | | |
| | WEIGHT | | | | | | |
| | REPS | | | | | | |
| | WEIGHT | | | | | | |
| | REPS | | | | | | |
| | WEIGHT | | | | | | |
| | REPS | | | | | | |
| | WEIGHT | | | | | | |
| | REPS | | | | | | |
| | WEIGHT | | | | | | |
| | REPS | | | | | | |
| | WEIGHT | | | | | | |
| | REPS | | | | | | |
| | WEIGHT | | | | | | |
| | REPS | | | | | | |
| | WEIGHT | | | | | | |
| | REPS | | | | | | |

**CARDIO ACTIVITY:**

**NOTES:**

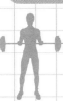

## TIP
Give yourself a pat on the back. You are taking better care of yourself.

# YOUR TRAINING JOURNAL

DATE

| EXERCISE | | SET 1 | SET 2 | SET 3 | SET 4 | SET 5 | SET 6 |
|---|---|---|---|---|---|---|---|
| | WEIGHT | | | | | | |
| | REPS | | | | | | |
| | WEIGHT | | | | | | |
| | REPS | | | | | | |
| | WEIGHT | | | | | | |
| | REPS | | | | | | |
| | WEIGHT | | | | | | |
| | REPS | | | | | | |
| | WEIGHT | | | | | | |
| | REPS | | | | | | |
| | WEIGHT | | | | | | |
| | REPS | | | | | | |
| | WEIGHT | | | | | | |
| | REPS | | | | | | |
| | WEIGHT | | | | | | |
| | REPS | | | | | | |
| | WEIGHT | | | | | | |
| | REPS | | | | | | |
| | WEIGHT | | | | | | |
| | REPS | | | | | | |
| | WEIGHT | | | | | | |
| | REPS | | | | | | |

**CARDIO ACTIVITY:**

**NOTES:**

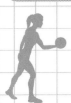

## TIP
Be careful with your body. If your body feels fatigued during your workout you could be overtraining.

# YOUR TRAINING
# JOURNAL

**DATE**

| EXERCISE | | SET 1 | SET 2 | SET 3 | SET 4 | SET 5 | SET 6 |
|---|---|---|---|---|---|---|---|
| | WEIGHT | | | | | | |
| | REPS | | | | | | |
| | WEIGHT | | | | | | |
| | REPS | | | | | | |
| | WEIGHT | | | | | | |
| | REPS | | | | | | |
| | WEIGHT | | | | | | |
| | REPS | | | | | | |
| | WEIGHT | | | | | | |
| | REPS | | | | | | |
| | WEIGHT | | | | | | |
| | REPS | | | | | | |
| | WEIGHT | | | | | | |
| | REPS | | | | | | |
| | WEIGHT | | | | | | |
| | REPS | | | | | | |
| | WEIGHT | | | | | | |
| | REPS | | | | | | |
| | WEIGHT | | | | | | |
| | REPS | | | | | | |
| | WEIGHT | | | | | | |
| | REPS | | | | | | |

**CARDIO ACTIVITY:**

**NOTES:**

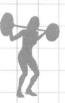

## TIP
Don't do anything else once you have convinced yourself
to go to the gym. Just go! You'll feel better.

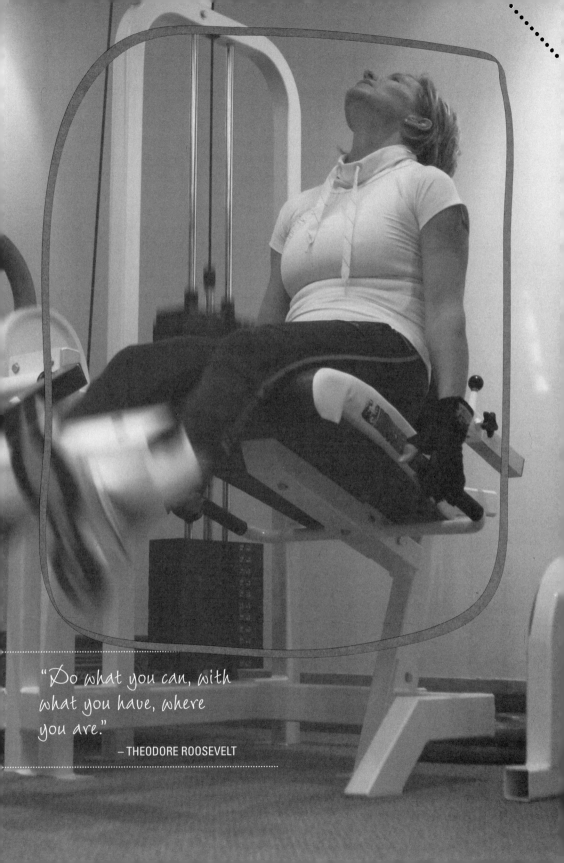

"Do what you can, with what you have, where you are."

— THEODORE ROOSEVELT

# YOUR TRAINING
# JOURNAL

DATE

| EXERCISE | | SET 1 | SET 2 | SET 3 | SET 4 | SET 5 | SET 6 |
|----------|--------|-------|-------|-------|-------|-------|-------|
| | WEIGHT | | | | | | |
| | REPS | | | | | | |
| | WEIGHT | | | | | | |
| | REPS | | | | | | |
| | WEIGHT | | | | | | |
| | REPS | | | | | | |
| | WEIGHT | | | | | | |
| | REPS | | | | | | |
| | WEIGHT | | | | | | |
| | REPS | | | | | | |
| | WEIGHT | | | | | | |
| | REPS | | | | | | |
| | WEIGHT | | | | | | |
| | REPS | | | | | | |
| | WEIGHT | | | | | | |
| | REPS | | | | | | |
| | WEIGHT | | | | | | |
| | REPS | | | | | | |
| | WEIGHT | | | | | | |
| | REPS | | | | | | |
| | WEIGHT | | | | | | |
| | REPS | | | | | | |

**CARDIO ACTIVITY:**

**NOTES:**

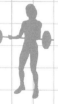

## TIP
Cool down after your workout. Stretch, breathe and let your heart get back to its normal pace.

# YOUR TRAINING
# JOURNAL

**DATE**

| EXERCISE | | SET 1 | SET 2 | SET 3 | SET 4 | SET 5 | SET 6 |
|---|---|---|---|---|---|---|---|
| | WEIGHT | | | | | | |
| | REPS | | | | | | |
| | WEIGHT | | | | | | |
| | REPS | | | | | | |
| | WEIGHT | | | | | | |
| | REPS | | | | | | |
| | WEIGHT | | | | | | |
| | REPS | | | | | | |
| | WEIGHT | | | | | | |
| | REPS | | | | | | |
| | WEIGHT | | | | | | |
| | REPS | | | | | | |
| | WEIGHT | | | | | | |
| | REPS | | | | | | |
| | WEIGHT | | | | | | |
| | REPS | | | | | | |
| | WEIGHT | | | | | | |
| | REPS | | | | | | |
| | WEIGHT | | | | | | |
| | REPS | | | | | | |
| | WEIGHT | | | | | | |
| | REPS | | | | | | |

**CARDIO ACTIVITY:**

**NOTES:**

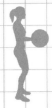

## TIP
Join an adult sports team to put your newly acquired fitness to the test.

# YOUR TRAINING
# JOURNAL

DATE

| EXERCISE | | SET 1 | SET 2 | SET 3 | SET 4 | SET 5 | SET 6 |
|---|---|---|---|---|---|---|---|
| | WEIGHT | | | | | | |
| | REPS | | | | | | |
| | WEIGHT | | | | | | |
| | REPS | | | | | | |
| | WEIGHT | | | | | | |
| | REPS | | | | | | |
| | WEIGHT | | | | | | |
| | REPS | | | | | | |
| | WEIGHT | | | | | | |
| | REPS | | | | | | |
| | WEIGHT | | | | | | |
| | REPS | | | | | | |
| | WEIGHT | | | | | | |
| | REPS | | | | | | |
| | WEIGHT | | | | | | |
| | REPS | | | | | | |
| | WEIGHT | | | | | | |
| | REPS | | | | | | |
| | WEIGHT | | | | | | |
| | REPS | | | | | | |
| | WEIGHT | | | | | | |
| | REPS | | | | | | |

**CARDIO ACTIVITY:**

**NOTES:**

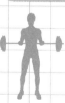

## TIP
Fulfill that childhood passion you had to dance, go blading or kayaking. Instead of movie night, try bowling or laser tag.

# YOUR TRAINING JOURNAL

DATE

| EXERCISE | | SET 1 | SET 2 | SET 3 | SET 4 | SET 5 | SET 6 |
|---|---|---|---|---|---|---|---|
| | WEIGHT | | | | | | |
| | REPS | | | | | | |
| | WEIGHT | | | | | | |
| | REPS | | | | | | |
| | WEIGHT | | | | | | |
| | REPS | | | | | | |
| | WEIGHT | | | | | | |
| | REPS | | | | | | |
| | WEIGHT | | | | | | |
| | REPS | | | | | | |
| | WEIGHT | | | | | | |
| | REPS | | | | | | |
| | WEIGHT | | | | | | |
| | REPS | | | | | | |
| | WEIGHT | | | | | | |
| | REPS | | | | | | |
| | WEIGHT | | | | | | |
| | REPS | | | | | | |
| | WEIGHT | | | | | | |
| | REPS | | | | | | |
| | WEIGHT | | | | | | |
| | REPS | | | | | | |

**CARDIO ACTIVITY:**

**NOTES:**

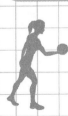

## TIP
Do cardio in the morning and weights later in the day to super charge your metabolism twice.

# YOUR TRAINING
# JOURNAL

DATE

| EXERCISE | | SET 1 | SET 2 | SET 3 | SET 4 | SET 5 | SET 6 |
|----------|---|-------|-------|-------|-------|-------|-------|
| | WEIGHT | | | | | | |
| | REPS | | | | | | |
| | WEIGHT | | | | | | |
| | REPS | | | | | | |
| | WEIGHT | | | | | | |
| | REPS | | | | | | |
| | WEIGHT | | | | | | |
| | REPS | | | | | | |
| | WEIGHT | | | | | | |
| | REPS | | | | | | |
| | WEIGHT | | | | | | |
| | REPS | | | | | | |
| | WEIGHT | | | | | | |
| | REPS | | | | | | |
| | WEIGHT | | | | | | |
| | REPS | | | | | | |
| | WEIGHT | | | | | | |
| | REPS | | | | | | |
| | WEIGHT | | | | | | |
| | REPS | | | | | | |
| | WEIGHT | | | | | | |
| | REPS | | | | | | |

**CARDIO ACTIVITY:**

**NOTES:**

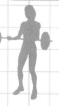

## TIP

Wear a heart-rate monitor to keep track of what your heart is doing while you train.

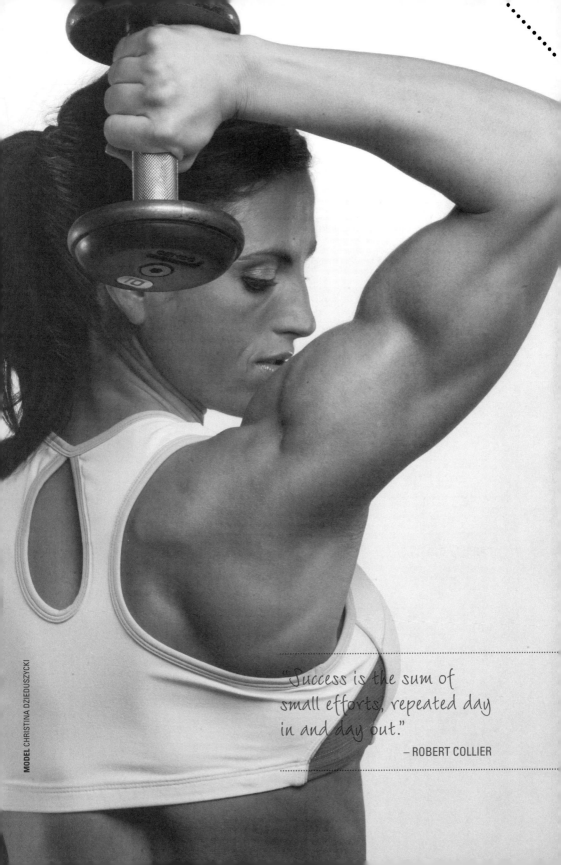

"Success is the sum of small efforts, repeated day in and day out."

– ROBERT COLLIER

# YOUR TRAINING
# JOURNAL

DATE

| EXERCISE | | SET 1 | SET 2 | SET 3 | SET 4 | SET 5 | SET 6 |
|---|---|---|---|---|---|---|---|
| | WEIGHT | | | | | | |
| | REPS | | | | | | |
| | WEIGHT | | | | | | |
| | REPS | | | | | | |
| | WEIGHT | | | | | | |
| | REPS | | | | | | |
| | WEIGHT | | | | | | |
| | REPS | | | | | | |
| | WEIGHT | | | | | | |
| | REPS | | | | | | |
| | WEIGHT | | | | | | |
| | REPS | | | | | | |
| | WEIGHT | | | | | | |
| | REPS | | | | | | |
| | WEIGHT | | | | | | |
| | REPS | | | | | | |
| | WEIGHT | | | | | | |
| | REPS | | | | | | |
| | WEIGHT | | | | | | |
| | REPS | | | | | | |
| | WEIGHT | | | | | | |
| | REPS | | | | | | |

**CARDIO ACTIVITY:**

**NOTES:**

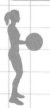

## TIP
In the early stages of training your job is basic — stick with no more than eight simple exercises.

# YOUR TRAINING JOURNAL

**DATE**

| EXERCISE | | SET 1 | SET 2 | SET 3 | SET 4 | SET 5 | SET 6 |
|---|---|---|---|---|---|---|---|
| | WEIGHT | | | | | | |
| | REPS | | | | | | |
| | WEIGHT | | | | | | |
| | REPS | | | | | | |
| | WEIGHT | | | | | | |
| | REPS | | | | | | |
| | WEIGHT | | | | | | |
| | REPS | | | | | | |
| | WEIGHT | | | | | | |
| | REPS | | | | | | |
| | WEIGHT | | | | | | |
| | REPS | | | | | | |
| | WEIGHT | | | | | | |
| | REPS | | | | | | |
| | WEIGHT | | | | | | |
| | REPS | | | | | | |
| | WEIGHT | | | | | | |
| | REPS | | | | | | |
| | WEIGHT | | | | | | |
| | REPS | | | | | | |
| | WEIGHT | | | | | | |
| | REPS | | | | | | |

**CARDIO ACTIVITY:**

**NOTES:**

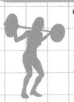

## TIP
Good clean nutrition, like good training, is simple. Learn the basics and practice them consistently.

# YOUR TRAINING JOURNAL

**DATE**

| EXERCISE | | SET 1 | SET 2 | SET 3 | SET 4 | SET 5 | SET 6 |
|---|---|---|---|---|---|---|---|
| | WEIGHT | | | | | | |
| | REPS | | | | | | |
| | WEIGHT | | | | | | |
| | REPS | | | | | | |
| | WEIGHT | | | | | | |
| | REPS | | | | | | |
| | WEIGHT | | | | | | |
| | REPS | | | | | | |
| | WEIGHT | | | | | | |
| | REPS | | | | | | |
| | WEIGHT | | | | | | |
| | REPS | | | | | | |
| | WEIGHT | | | | | | |
| | REPS | | | | | | |
| | WEIGHT | | | | | | |
| | REPS | | | | | | |
| | WEIGHT | | | | | | |
| | REPS | | | | | | |
| | WEIGHT | | | | | | |
| | REPS | | | | | | |
| | WEIGHT | | | | | | |
| | REPS | | | | | | |

**CARDIO ACTIVITY:**

**NOTES:**

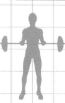

## TIP

Don't forget to eat 6 small meals each day. Eat every 2 to 3 hours for maximum fat burning.

# YOUR TRAINING JOURNAL

DATE

| EXERCISE | | SET 1 | SET 2 | SET 3 | SET 4 | SET 5 | SET 6 |
|---|---|---|---|---|---|---|---|
| | WEIGHT | | | | | | |
| | REPS | | | | | | |
| | WEIGHT | | | | | | |
| | REPS | | | | | | |
| | WEIGHT | | | | | | |
| | REPS | | | | | | |
| | WEIGHT | | | | | | |
| | REPS | | | | | | |
| | WEIGHT | | | | | | |
| | REPS | | | | | | |
| | WEIGHT | | | | | | |
| | REPS | | | | | | |
| | WEIGHT | | | | | | |
| | REPS | | | | | | |
| | WEIGHT | | | | | | |
| | REPS | | | | | | |
| | WEIGHT | | | | | | |
| | REPS | | | | | | |
| | WEIGHT | | | | | | |
| | REPS | | | | | | |
| | WEIGHT | | | | | | |
| | REPS | | | | | | |

**CARDIO ACTIVITY:**

**NOTES:**

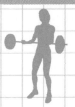

## TIP
If you have a fondness for alcohol that is ruining your life, stop drinking. Get help and start training and Eating Clean today.

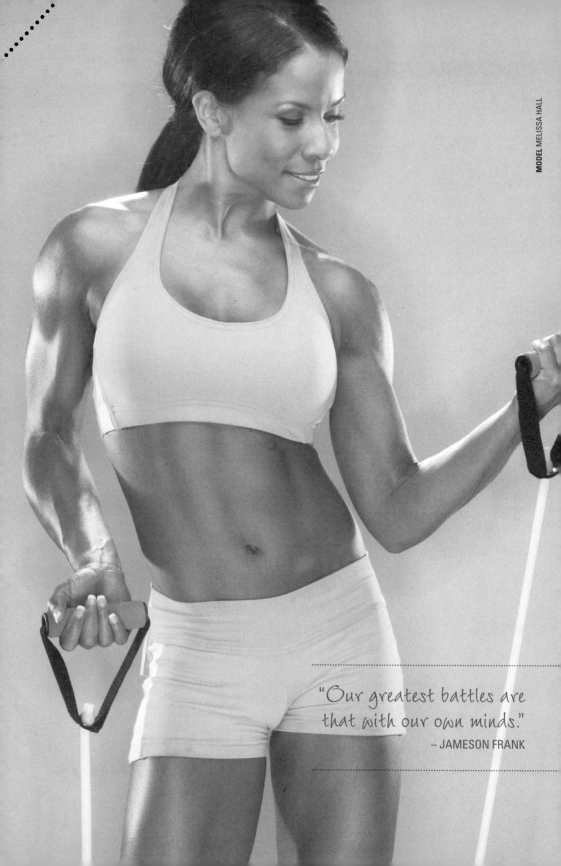

"Our greatest battles are
that with our own minds."
– JAMESON FRANK

# YOUR TRAINING JOURNAL

**DATE**

| EXERCISE | | SET 1 | SET 2 | SET 3 | SET 4 | SET 5 | SET 6 |
|---|---|---|---|---|---|---|---|
| | WEIGHT | | | | | | |
| | REPS | | | | | | |
| | WEIGHT | | | | | | |
| | REPS | | | | | | |
| | WEIGHT | | | | | | |
| | REPS | | | | | | |
| | WEIGHT | | | | | | |
| | REPS | | | | | | |
| | WEIGHT | | | | | | |
| | REPS | | | | | | |
| | WEIGHT | | | | | | |
| | REPS | | | | | | |
| | WEIGHT | | | | | | |
| | REPS | | | | | | |
| | WEIGHT | | | | | | |
| | REPS | | | | | | |
| | WEIGHT | | | | | | |
| | REPS | | | | | | |
| | WEIGHT | | | | | | |
| | REPS | | | | | | |
| | WEIGHT | | | | | | |
| | REPS | | | | | | |

**CARDIO ACTIVITY:**

**NOTES:**

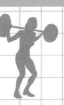

## TIP
We all have doubts about our appearance, abilities, strengths and weaknesses. Regardless of your insecurities, decide to be the best you can be.

# YOUR TRAINING JOURNAL

DATE

| EXERCISE | | SET 1 | SET 2 | SET 3 | SET 4 | SET 5 | SET 6 |
|---|---|---|---|---|---|---|---|
| | WEIGHT | | | | | | |
| | REPS | | | | | | |
| | WEIGHT | | | | | | |
| | REPS | | | | | | |
| | WEIGHT | | | | | | |
| | REPS | | | | | | |
| | WEIGHT | | | | | | |
| | REPS | | | | | | |
| | WEIGHT | | | | | | |
| | REPS | | | | | | |
| | WEIGHT | | | | | | |
| | REPS | | | | | | |
| | WEIGHT | | | | | | |
| | REPS | | | | | | |
| | WEIGHT | | | | | | |
| | REPS | | | | | | |
| | WEIGHT | | | | | | |
| | REPS | | | | | | |
| | WEIGHT | | | | | | |
| | REPS | | | | | | |
| | WEIGHT | | | | | | |
| | REPS | | | | | | |

**CARDIO ACTIVITY:**

**NOTES:**

## TIP

When setting up a home gym, define your workout area in the garage, bedroom or basement. Give yourself enough room to have a comfortable workout.

# YOUR TRAINING JOURNAL

DATE

| EXERCISE | | SET 1 | SET 2 | SET 3 | SET 4 | SET 5 | SET 6 |
|---|---|---|---|---|---|---|---|
| | WEIGHT | | | | | | |
| | REPS | | | | | | |
| | WEIGHT | | | | | | |
| | REPS | | | | | | |
| | WEIGHT | | | | | | |
| | REPS | | | | | | |
| | WEIGHT | | | | | | |
| | REPS | | | | | | |
| | WEIGHT | | | | | | |
| | REPS | | | | | | |
| | WEIGHT | | | | | | |
| | REPS | | | | | | |
| | WEIGHT | | | | | | |
| | REPS | | | | | | |
| | WEIGHT | | | | | | |
| | REPS | | | | | | |
| | WEIGHT | | | | | | |
| | REPS | | | | | | |
| | WEIGHT | | | | | | |
| | REPS | | | | | | |
| | WEIGHT | | | | | | |
| | REPS | | | | | | |

**CARDIO ACTIVITY:**

**NOTES:**

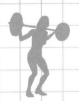

## TIP
Include stretching after a workout when muscles are warm. This helps to prevent injury.

# YOUR TRAINING JOURNAL

**DATE**

| EXERCISE | | SET 1 | SET 2 | SET 3 | SET 4 | SET 5 | SET 6 |
|---|---|---|---|---|---|---|---|
| | WEIGHT | | | | | | |
| | REPS | | | | | | |
| | WEIGHT | | | | | | |
| | REPS | | | | | | |
| | WEIGHT | | | | | | |
| | REPS | | | | | | |
| | WEIGHT | | | | | | |
| | REPS | | | | | | |
| | WEIGHT | | | | | | |
| | REPS | | | | | | |
| | WEIGHT | | | | | | |
| | REPS | | | | | | |
| | WEIGHT | | | | | | |
| | REPS | | | | | | |
| | WEIGHT | | | | | | |
| | REPS | | | | | | |
| | WEIGHT | | | | | | |
| | REPS | | | | | | |
| | WEIGHT | | | | | | |
| | REPS | | | | | | |
| | WEIGHT | | | | | | |
| | REPS | | | | | | |

**CARDIO ACTIVITY:**

**NOTES:**

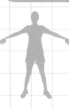

## TIP
Attend a yoga class every so often to keep limber and calm.

# YOUR TRAINING JOURNAL

DATE

| EXERCISE | | SET 1 | SET 2 | SET 3 | SET 4 | SET 5 | SET 6 |
|---|---|---|---|---|---|---|---|
| | WEIGHT | | | | | | |
| | REPS | | | | | | |
| | WEIGHT | | | | | | |
| | REPS | | | | | | |
| | WEIGHT | | | | | | |
| | REPS | | | | | | |
| | WEIGHT | | | | | | |
| | REPS | | | | | | |
| | WEIGHT | | | | | | |
| | REPS | | | | | | |
| | WEIGHT | | | | | | |
| | REPS | | | | | | |
| | WEIGHT | | | | | | |
| | REPS | | | | | | |
| | WEIGHT | | | | | | |
| | REPS | | | | | | |
| | WEIGHT | | | | | | |
| | REPS | | | | | | |
| | WEIGHT | | | | | | |
| | REPS | | | | | | |
| | WEIGHT | | | | | | |
| | REPS | | | | | | |

**CARDIO ACTIVITY:**

**NOTES:**

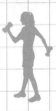

## TIP

Vary your workouts. Instead of a run, go for a high-energy salsa class or jump on a mountain bike.

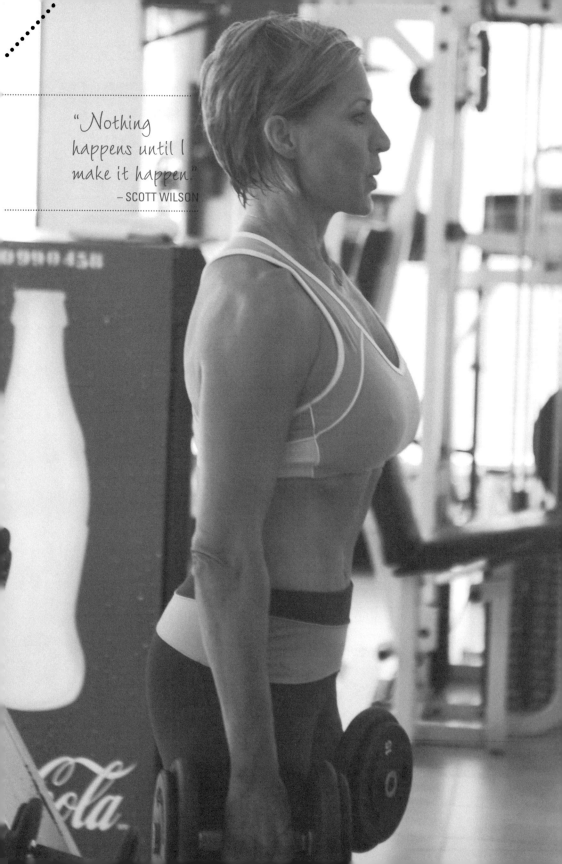

"Nothing
happens until I
make it happen."
– SCOTT WILSON

# YOUR TRAINING JOURNAL

DATE

| EXERCISE | | SET 1 | SET 2 | SET 3 | SET 4 | SET 5 | SET 6 |
|---|---|---|---|---|---|---|---|
| | WEIGHT | | | | | | |
| | REPS | | | | | | |
| | WEIGHT | | | | | | |
| | REPS | | | | | | |
| | WEIGHT | | | | | | |
| | REPS | | | | | | |
| | WEIGHT | | | | | | |
| | REPS | | | | | | |
| | WEIGHT | | | | | | |
| | REPS | | | | | | |
| | WEIGHT | | | | | | |
| | REPS | | | | | | |
| | WEIGHT | | | | | | |
| | REPS | | | | | | |
| | WEIGHT | | | | | | |
| | REPS | | | | | | |
| | WEIGHT | | | | | | |
| | REPS | | | | | | |
| | WEIGHT | | | | | | |
| | REPS | | | | | | |
| | WEIGHT | | | | | | |
| | REPS | | | | | | |

**CARDIO ACTIVITY:**

**NOTES:**

## TIP
Make workout time family time. Go for a hike, swim, roller blade, skate, ski or bike ride together.

# YOUR TRAINING JOURNAL

**DATE** 

| EXERCISE | | SET 1 | SET 2 | SET 3 | SET 4 | SET 5 | SET 6 |
|---|---|---|---|---|---|---|---|
| | WEIGHT | | | | | | |
| | REPS | | | | | | |
| | WEIGHT | | | | | | |
| | REPS | | | | | | |
| | WEIGHT | | | | | | |
| | REPS | | | | | | |
| | WEIGHT | | | | | | |
| | REPS | | | | | | |
| | WEIGHT | | | | | | |
| | REPS | | | | | | |
| | WEIGHT | | | | | | |
| | REPS | | | | | | |
| | WEIGHT | | | | | | |
| | REPS | | | | | | |
| | WEIGHT | | | | | | |
| | REPS | | | | | | |
| | WEIGHT | | | | | | |
| | REPS | | | | | | |
| | WEIGHT | | | | | | |
| | REPS | | | | | | |
| | WEIGHT | | | | | | |
| | REPS | | | | | | |

**CARDIO ACTIVITY:**

**NOTES:**

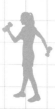

## TIP

Update your workout clothes. Get bright colors to keep you happy during your workout. Don't put your workout wear in the dryer.

# YOUR TRAINING JOURNAL

**DATE**

| EXERCISE | | SET 1 | SET 2 | SET 3 | SET 4 | SET 5 | SET 6 |
|---|---|---|---|---|---|---|---|
| | WEIGHT | | | | | | |
| | REPS | | | | | | |
| | WEIGHT | | | | | | |
| | REPS | | | | | | |
| | WEIGHT | | | | | | |
| | REPS | | | | | | |
| | WEIGHT | | | | | | |
| | REPS | | | | | | |
| | WEIGHT | | | | | | |
| | REPS | | | | | | |
| | WEIGHT | | | | | | |
| | REPS | | | | | | |
| | WEIGHT | | | | | | |
| | REPS | | | | | | |
| | WEIGHT | | | | | | |
| | REPS | | | | | | |
| | WEIGHT | | | | | | |
| | REPS | | | | | | |
| | WEIGHT | | | | | | |
| | REPS | | | | | | |
| | WEIGHT | | | | | | |
| | REPS | | | | | | |

**CARDIO ACTIVITY:**

**NOTES:**

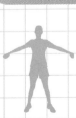

## TIP
Organize a group run or walk for coworkers at your place of work during lunch hour.

# YOUR TRAINING
# JOURNAL

**DATE**

| EXERCISE | | SET 1 | SET 2 | SET 3 | SET 4 | SET 5 | SET 6 |
|---|---|---|---|---|---|---|---|
| | WEIGHT | | | | | | |
| | REPS | | | | | | |
| | WEIGHT | | | | | | |
| | REPS | | | | | | |
| | WEIGHT | | | | | | |
| | REPS | | | | | | |
| | WEIGHT | | | | | | |
| | REPS | | | | | | |
| | WEIGHT | | | | | | |
| | REPS | | | | | | |
| | WEIGHT | | | | | | |
| | REPS | | | | | | |
| | WEIGHT | | | | | | |
| | REPS | | | | | | |
| | WEIGHT | | | | | | |
| | REPS | | | | | | |
| | WEIGHT | | | | | | |
| | REPS | | | | | | |
| | WEIGHT | | | | | | |
| | REPS | | | | | | |
| | WEIGHT | | | | | | |
| | REPS | | | | | | |

**CARDIO ACTIVITY:**

**NOTES:**

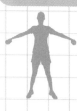

## TIP
Enter a competition to give yourself a goal to work toward.

# YOUR TRAINING
# JOURNAL

DATE

| EXERCISE | | SET 1 | SET 2 | SET 3 | SET 4 | SET 5 | SET 6 |
|---|---|---|---|---|---|---|---|
| | WEIGHT | | | | | | |
| | REPS | | | | | | |
| | WEIGHT | | | | | | |
| | REPS | | | | | | |
| | WEIGHT | | | | | | |
| | REPS | | | | | | |
| | WEIGHT | | | | | | |
| | REPS | | | | | | |
| | WEIGHT | | | | | | |
| | REPS | | | | | | |
| | WEIGHT | | | | | | |
| | REPS | | | | | | |
| | WEIGHT | | | | | | |
| | REPS | | | | | | |
| | WEIGHT | | | | | | |
| | REPS | | | | | | |
| | WEIGHT | | | | | | |
| | REPS | | | | | | |
| | WEIGHT | | | | | | |
| | REPS | | | | | | |
| | WEIGHT | | | | | | |
| | REPS | | | | | | |

**CARDIO ACTIVITY:**

**NOTES:**

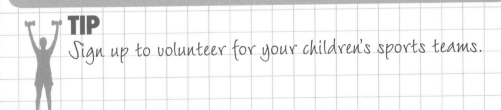

**TIP**
Sign up to volunteer for your children's sports teams.

# YOUR TRAINING
# JOURNAL

**DATE**

| EXERCISE | | SET 1 | SET 2 | SET 3 | SET 4 | SET 5 | SET 6 |
|---|---|---|---|---|---|---|---|
| | WEIGHT | | | | | | |
| | REPS | | | | | | |
| | WEIGHT | | | | | | |
| | REPS | | | | | | |
| | WEIGHT | | | | | | |
| | REPS | | | | | | |
| | WEIGHT | | | | | | |
| | REPS | | | | | | |
| | WEIGHT | | | | | | |
| | REPS | | | | | | |
| | WEIGHT | | | | | | |
| | REPS | | | | | | |
| | WEIGHT | | | | | | |
| | REPS | | | | | | |
| | WEIGHT | | | | | | |
| | REPS | | | | | | |
| | WEIGHT | | | | | | |
| | REPS | | | | | | |
| | WEIGHT | | | | | | |
| | REPS | | | | | | |
| | WEIGHT | | | | | | |
| | REPS | | | | | | |

**CARDIO ACTIVITY:**

**NOTES:**

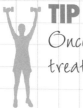

**TIP**

Once you have achieved a workout goal, buy yourself a treat. Reward your efforts with a non-food goody.

"Our best success comes
after our greatest
disappointments."
— HENRY WARD BEECHER

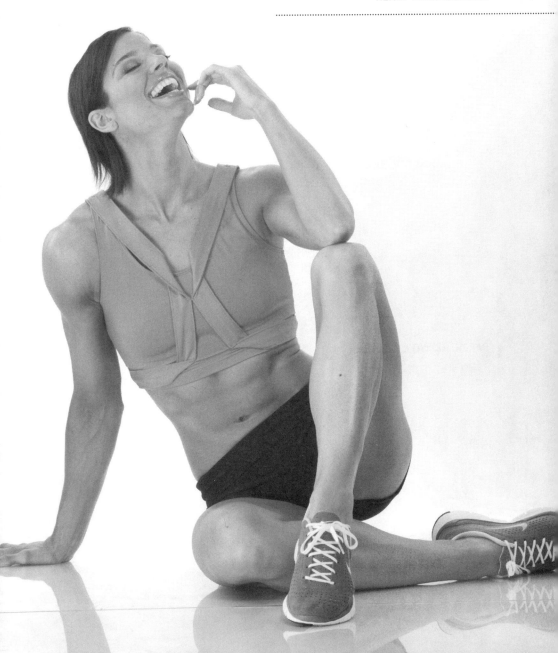

# YOUR TRAINING
# JOURNAL

**DATE** [ ]

| EXERCISE | | SET 1 | SET 2 | SET 3 | SET 4 | SET 5 | SET 6 |
|---|---|---|---|---|---|---|---|
| | WEIGHT | | | | | | |
| | REPS | | | | | | |
| | WEIGHT | | | | | | |
| | REPS | | | | | | |
| | WEIGHT | | | | | | |
| | REPS | | | | | | |
| | WEIGHT | | | | | | |
| | REPS | | | | | | |
| | WEIGHT | | | | | | |
| | REPS | | | | | | |
| | WEIGHT | | | | | | |
| | REPS | | | | | | |
| | WEIGHT | | | | | | |
| | REPS | | | | | | |
| | WEIGHT | | | | | | |
| | REPS | | | | | | |
| | WEIGHT | | | | | | |
| | REPS | | | | | | |
| | WEIGHT | | | | | | |
| | REPS | | | | | | |
| | WEIGHT | | | | | | |
| | REPS | | | | | | |

**CARDIO ACTIVITY:**

**NOTES:**

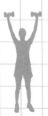

## TIP

Join a support system. An online blog like the one found on my forum is chock full of people doing the same thing as you. You can support each other. Visit www.toscareno.com.

# YOUR TRAINING JOURNAL

DATE

| EXERCISE | | SET 1 | SET 2 | SET 3 | SET 4 | SET 5 | SET 6 |
|---|---|---|---|---|---|---|---|
| | WEIGHT | | | | | | |
| | REPS | | | | | | |
| | WEIGHT | | | | | | |
| | REPS | | | | | | |
| | WEIGHT | | | | | | |
| | REPS | | | | | | |
| | WEIGHT | | | | | | |
| | REPS | | | | | | |
| | WEIGHT | | | | | | |
| | REPS | | | | | | |
| | WEIGHT | | | | | | |
| | REPS | | | | | | |
| | WEIGHT | | | | | | |
| | REPS | | | | | | |
| | WEIGHT | | | | | | |
| | REPS | | | | | | |
| | WEIGHT | | | | | | |
| | REPS | | | | | | |
| | WEIGHT | | | | | | |
| | REPS | | | | | | |
| | WEIGHT | | | | | | |
| | REPS | | | | | | |

**CARDIO ACTIVITY:**

**NOTES:**

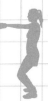

## TIP
Invent a family Friday night Dance Party. Ask your neighbors over and get your groove on.

# YOUR TRAINING JOURNAL

DATE

| EXERCISE | | SET 1 | SET 2 | SET 3 | SET 4 | SET 5 | SET 6 |
|---|---|---|---|---|---|---|---|
| | WEIGHT | | | | | | |
| | REPS | | | | | | |
| | WEIGHT | | | | | | |
| | REPS | | | | | | |
| | WEIGHT | | | | | | |
| | REPS | | | | | | |
| | WEIGHT | | | | | | |
| | REPS | | | | | | |
| | WEIGHT | | | | | | |
| | REPS | | | | | | |
| | WEIGHT | | | | | | |
| | REPS | | | | | | |
| | WEIGHT | | | | | | |
| | REPS | | | | | | |
| | WEIGHT | | | | | | |
| | REPS | | | | | | |
| | WEIGHT | | | | | | |
| | REPS | | | | | | |
| | WEIGHT | | | | | | |
| | REPS | | | | | | |
| | WEIGHT | | | | | | |
| | REPS | | | | | | |

**CARDIO ACTIVITY:**

**NOTES:**

## TIP

Go running in the rain while listening to Natasha Bedingfield's *Unwritten* on your iPod. It is liberating.

# YOUR TRAINING JOURNAL

**DATE**

| EXERCISE | | SET 1 | SET 2 | SET 3 | SET 4 | SET 5 | SET 6 |
|---|---|---|---|---|---|---|---|
| | WEIGHT | | | | | | |
| | REPS | | | | | | |
| | WEIGHT | | | | | | |
| | REPS | | | | | | |
| | WEIGHT | | | | | | |
| | REPS | | | | | | |
| | WEIGHT | | | | | | |
| | REPS | | | | | | |
| | WEIGHT | | | | | | |
| | REPS | | | | | | |
| | WEIGHT | | | | | | |
| | REPS | | | | | | |
| | WEIGHT | | | | | | |
| | REPS | | | | | | |
| | WEIGHT | | | | | | |
| | REPS | | | | | | |
| | WEIGHT | | | | | | |
| | REPS | | | | | | |
| | WEIGHT | | | | | | |
| | REPS | | | | | | |
| | WEIGHT | | | | | | |
| | REPS | | | | | | |

**CARDIO ACTIVITY:**

**NOTES:**

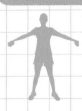

## TIP
Train with a friend or your special someone for a 5K, 10K or marathon.

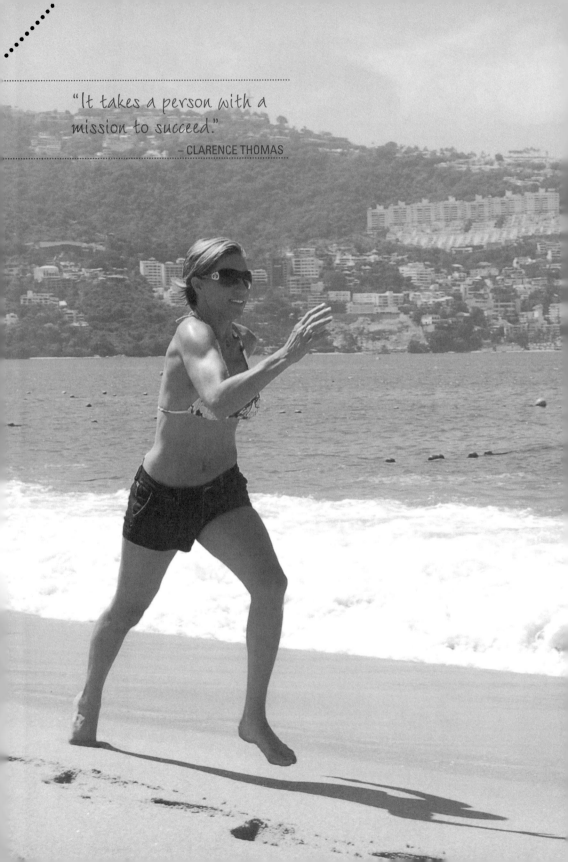

"It takes a person with a mission to succeed."
— CLARENCE THOMAS

# YOUR TRAINING JOURNAL

**DATE**

| EXERCISE | | SET 1 | SET 2 | SET 3 | SET 4 | SET 5 | SET 6 |
|---|---|---|---|---|---|---|---|
| | WEIGHT | | | | | | |
| | REPS | | | | | | |
| | WEIGHT | | | | | | |
| | REPS | | | | | | |
| | WEIGHT | | | | | | |
| | REPS | | | | | | |
| | WEIGHT | | | | | | |
| | REPS | | | | | | |
| | WEIGHT | | | | | | |
| | REPS | | | | | | |
| | WEIGHT | | | | | | |
| | REPS | | | | | | |
| | WEIGHT | | | | | | |
| | REPS | | | | | | |
| | WEIGHT | | | | | | |
| | REPS | | | | | | |
| | WEIGHT | | | | | | |
| | REPS | | | | | | |
| | WEIGHT | | | | | | |
| | REPS | | | | | | |
| | WEIGHT | | | | | | |
| | REPS | | | | | | |

**CARDIO ACTIVITY:**

**NOTES:**

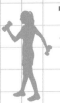

**TIP**
Treat yourself to a deep-tissue massage.

# YOUR TRAINING JOURNAL

**DATE**

| EXERCISE | | SET 1 | SET 2 | SET 3 | SET 4 | SET 5 | SET 6 |
|---|---|---|---|---|---|---|---|
| | WEIGHT | | | | | | |
| | REPS | | | | | | |
| | WEIGHT | | | | | | |
| | REPS | | | | | | |
| | WEIGHT | | | | | | |
| | REPS | | | | | | |
| | WEIGHT | | | | | | |
| | REPS | | | | | | |
| | WEIGHT | | | | | | |
| | REPS | | | | | | |
| | WEIGHT | | | | | | |
| | REPS | | | | | | |
| | WEIGHT | | | | | | |
| | REPS | | | | | | |
| | WEIGHT | | | | | | |
| | REPS | | | | | | |
| | WEIGHT | | | | | | |
| | REPS | | | | | | |
| | WEIGHT | | | | | | |
| | REPS | | | | | | |
| | WEIGHT | | | | | | |
| | REPS | | | | | | |

**CARDIO ACTIVITY:**

**NOTES:**

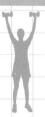

## TIP
Go into your workout with a positive, happy attitude.
Tell yourself this is going to be the best workout ever.

# YOUR TRAINING
# JOURNAL

**DATE**

| EXERCISE | | SET 1 | SET 2 | SET 3 | SET 4 | SET 5 | SET 6 |
|---|---|---|---|---|---|---|---|
| | WEIGHT | | | | | | |
| | REPS | | | | | | |
| | WEIGHT | | | | | | |
| | REPS | | | | | | |
| | WEIGHT | | | | | | |
| | REPS | | | | | | |
| | WEIGHT | | | | | | |
| | REPS | | | | | | |
| | WEIGHT | | | | | | |
| | REPS | | | | | | |
| | WEIGHT | | | | | | |
| | REPS | | | | | | |
| | WEIGHT | | | | | | |
| | REPS | | | | | | |
| | WEIGHT | | | | | | |
| | REPS | | | | | | |
| | WEIGHT | | | | | | |
| | REPS | | | | | | |
| | WEIGHT | | | | | | |
| | REPS | | | | | | |
| | WEIGHT | | | | | | |
| | REPS | | | | | | |

**CARDIO ACTIVITY:**

**NOTES:**

## TIP
Have a Clean-Eating snack when your workout is done.

# YOUR TRAINING
# JOURNAL

DATE

| EXERCISE | | SET 1 | SET 2 | SET 3 | SET 4 | SET 5 | SET 6 |
|---|---|---|---|---|---|---|---|
| | WEIGHT | | | | | | |
| | REPS | | | | | | |
| | WEIGHT | | | | | | |
| | REPS | | | | | | |
| | WEIGHT | | | | | | |
| | REPS | | | | | | |
| | WEIGHT | | | | | | |
| | REPS | | | | | | |
| | WEIGHT | | | | | | |
| | REPS | | | | | | |
| | WEIGHT | | | | | | |
| | REPS | | | | | | |
| | WEIGHT | | | | | | |
| | REPS | | | | | | |
| | WEIGHT | | | | | | |
| | REPS | | | | | | |
| | WEIGHT | | | | | | |
| | REPS | | | | | | |
| | WEIGHT | | | | | | |
| | REPS | | | | | | |
| | WEIGHT | | | | | | |
| | REPS | | | | | | |

**CARDIO ACTIVITY:**

**NOTES:**

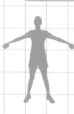

## TIP
Go for a Mystic Tan®. This spray-on tan will give your skin a gorgeous glow and make you look five pounds slimmer.

# YOUR TRAINING JOURNAL

**DATE**

| EXERCISE | | SET 1 | SET 2 | SET 3 | SET 4 | SET 5 | SET 6 |
|---|---|---|---|---|---|---|---|
| | WEIGHT | | | | | | |
| | REPS | | | | | | |
| | WEIGHT | | | | | | |
| | REPS | | | | | | |
| | WEIGHT | | | | | | |
| | REPS | | | | | | |
| | WEIGHT | | | | | | |
| | REPS | | | | | | |
| | WEIGHT | | | | | | |
| | REPS | | | | | | |
| | WEIGHT | | | | | | |
| | REPS | | | | | | |
| | WEIGHT | | | | | | |
| | REPS | | | | | | |
| | WEIGHT | | | | | | |
| | REPS | | | | | | |
| | WEIGHT | | | | | | |
| | REPS | | | | | | |
| | WEIGHT | | | | | | |
| | REPS | | | | | | |
| | WEIGHT | | | | | | |
| | REPS | | | | | | |

**CARDIO ACTIVITY:**

**NOTES:**

## TIP

Pain and injury, though not our chosen friends, serve us well in lessons learned. Take care with your training; never fail to warm up properly.

# YOUR TRAINING
# JOURNAL

**DATE**

| EXERCISE | | SET 1 | SET 2 | SET 3 | SET 4 | SET 5 | SET 6 |
|----------|--|-------|-------|-------|-------|-------|-------|
| | WEIGHT | | | | | | |
| | REPS | | | | | | |
| | WEIGHT | | | | | | |
| | REPS | | | | | | |
| | WEIGHT | | | | | | |
| | REPS | | | | | | |
| | WEIGHT | | | | | | |
| | REPS | | | | | | |
| | WEIGHT | | | | | | |
| | REPS | | | | | | |
| | WEIGHT | | | | | | |
| | REPS | | | | | | |
| | WEIGHT | | | | | | |
| | REPS | | | | | | |
| | WEIGHT | | | | | | |
| | REPS | | | | | | |
| | WEIGHT | | | | | | |
| | REPS | | | | | | |
| | WEIGHT | | | | | | |
| | REPS | | | | | | |
| | WEIGHT | | | | | | |
| | REPS | | | | | | |

**CARDIO ACTIVITY:**

**NOTES:**

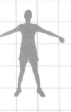

## TIP

Don't let change sabotage your efforts. Your training partner fails to show. Your job changes. The kids need a ride. Your mother is feeling poorly. Soldier on. Fit in your training regardless.

"Set your goals high, and don't stop till you get there."

– BO JACKSON

# YOUR TRAINING JOURNAL

DATE

| EXERCISE | | SET 1 | SET 2 | SET 3 | SET 4 | SET 5 | SET 6 |
|---|---|---|---|---|---|---|---|
| | WEIGHT | | | | | | |
| | REPS | | | | | | |
| | WEIGHT | | | | | | |
| | REPS | | | | | | |
| | WEIGHT | | | | | | |
| | REPS | | | | | | |
| | WEIGHT | | | | | | |
| | REPS | | | | | | |
| | WEIGHT | | | | | | |
| | REPS | | | | | | |
| | WEIGHT | | | | | | |
| | REPS | | | | | | |
| | WEIGHT | | | | | | |
| | REPS | | | | | | |
| | WEIGHT | | | | | | |
| | REPS | | | | | | |
| | WEIGHT | | | | | | |
| | REPS | | | | | | |
| | WEIGHT | | | | | | |
| | REPS | | | | | | |
| | WEIGHT | | | | | | |
| | REPS | | | | | | |

**CARDIO ACTIVITY:**

**NOTES:**

 **TIP**

If you smoke stop now. No second thoughts, just do it!
Cigarettes dig into your health like rusty nails.

# YOUR TRAINING JOURNAL

DATE

| EXERCISE | | SET 1 | SET 2 | SET 3 | SET 4 | SET 5 | SET 6 |
|---|---|---|---|---|---|---|---|
| | WEIGHT | | | | | | |
| | REPS | | | | | | |
| | WEIGHT | | | | | | |
| | REPS | | | | | | |
| | WEIGHT | | | | | | |
| | REPS | | | | | | |
| | WEIGHT | | | | | | |
| | REPS | | | | | | |
| | WEIGHT | | | | | | |
| | REPS | | | | | | |
| | WEIGHT | | | | | | |
| | REPS | | | | | | |
| | WEIGHT | | | | | | |
| | REPS | | | | | | |
| | WEIGHT | | | | | | |
| | REPS | | | | | | |
| | WEIGHT | | | | | | |
| | REPS | | | | | | |
| | WEIGHT | | | | | | |
| | REPS | | | | | | |
| | WEIGHT | | | | | | |
| | REPS | | | | | | |

**CARDIO ACTIVITY:**

**NOTES:**

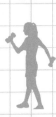

## TIP
Results come quickly to the beginner. But in time things appear to come to a screeching halt. Be confident that if you stick to the basics, progress is always taking place.

# YOUR TRAINING JOURNAL

**DATE** [      ]

| EXERCISE | | SET 1 | SET 2 | SET 3 | SET 4 | SET 5 | SET 6 |
|---|---|---|---|---|---|---|---|
| | WEIGHT | | | | | | |
| | REPS | | | | | | |
| | WEIGHT | | | | | | |
| | REPS | | | | | | |
| | WEIGHT | | | | | | |
| | REPS | | | | | | |
| | WEIGHT | | | | | | |
| | REPS | | | | | | |
| | WEIGHT | | | | | | |
| | REPS | | | | | | |
| | WEIGHT | | | | | | |
| | REPS | | | | | | |
| | WEIGHT | | | | | | |
| | REPS | | | | | | |
| | WEIGHT | | | | | | |
| | REPS | | | | | | |
| | WEIGHT | | | | | | |
| | REPS | | | | | | |
| | WEIGHT | | | | | | |
| | REPS | | | | | | |
| | WEIGHT | | | | | | |
| | REPS | | | | | | |

**CARDIO ACTIVITY:**

**NOTES:**

## TIP

Feel shaky during a workout? You may be training too intensely, in which case you need to slow down or use lighter weights. Make sure to eat for energy before training. A banana and yogurt will do.

# YOUR TRAINING
# JOURNAL

**DATE**

| EXERCISE | | SET 1 | SET 2 | SET 3 | SET 4 | SET 5 | SET 6 |
|---|---|---|---|---|---|---|---|
| | WEIGHT | | | | | | |
| | REPS | | | | | | |
| | WEIGHT | | | | | | |
| | REPS | | | | | | |
| | WEIGHT | | | | | | |
| | REPS | | | | | | |
| | WEIGHT | | | | | | |
| | REPS | | | | | | |
| | WEIGHT | | | | | | |
| | REPS | | | | | | |
| | WEIGHT | | | | | | |
| | REPS | | | | | | |
| | WEIGHT | | | | | | |
| | REPS | | | | | | |
| | WEIGHT | | | | | | |
| | REPS | | | | | | |
| | WEIGHT | | | | | | |
| | REPS | | | | | | |
| | WEIGHT | | | | | | |
| | REPS | | | | | | |
| | WEIGHT | | | | | | |
| | REPS | | | | | | |

**CARDIO ACTIVITY:**

**NOTES:**

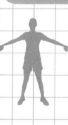

## TIP

Stand tall with abdominal muscles pulled in. Keeping your abs flexed throughout the day will cause them to stay firm even when you are relaxed, through a phenomenon called muscle memory.

# YOUR TRAINING
# JOURNAL

DATE

| EXERCISE | | SET 1 | SET 2 | SET 3 | SET 4 | SET 5 | SET 6 |
|---|---|---|---|---|---|---|---|
| | WEIGHT | | | | | | |
| | REPS | | | | | | |
| | WEIGHT | | | | | | |
| | REPS | | | | | | |
| | WEIGHT | | | | | | |
| | REPS | | | | | | |
| | WEIGHT | | | | | | |
| | REPS | | | | | | |
| | WEIGHT | | | | | | |
| | REPS | | | | | | |
| | WEIGHT | | | | | | |
| | REPS | | | | | | |
| | WEIGHT | | | | | | |
| | REPS | | | | | | |
| | WEIGHT | | | | | | |
| | REPS | | | | | | |
| | WEIGHT | | | | | | |
| | REPS | | | | | | |
| | WEIGHT | | | | | | |
| | REPS | | | | | | |
| | WEIGHT | | | | | | |
| | REPS | | | | | | |

**CARDIO ACTIVITY:**

**NOTES:**

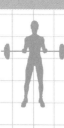

## TIP
Eat a combination of lean protein and complex carbohydrates from fresh fruit and vegetables and whole grains.

# YOUR TRAINING JOURNAL

DATE

| EXERCISE | | SET 1 | SET 2 | SET 3 | SET 4 | SET 5 | SET 6 |
|---|---|---|---|---|---|---|---|
| | WEIGHT | | | | | | |
| | REPS | | | | | | |
| | WEIGHT | | | | | | |
| | REPS | | | | | | |
| | WEIGHT | | | | | | |
| | REPS | | | | | | |
| | WEIGHT | | | | | | |
| | REPS | | | | | | |
| | WEIGHT | | | | | | |
| | REPS | | | | | | |
| | WEIGHT | | | | | | |
| | REPS | | | | | | |
| | WEIGHT | | | | | | |
| | REPS | | | | | | |
| | WEIGHT | | | | | | |
| | REPS | | | | | | |
| | WEIGHT | | | | | | |
| | REPS | | | | | | |
| | WEIGHT | | | | | | |
| | REPS | | | | | | |
| | WEIGHT | | | | | | |
| | REPS | | | | | | |

**CARDIO ACTIVITY:**

**NOTES:**

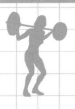

## TIP

Processed foods are imposters. They often contain chemical calories that sabotage your clean nutrition. Stick to foods you can readily recognize.

# YOUR TRAINING JOURNAL

**DATE**

| EXERCISE | | SET 1 | SET 2 | SET 3 | SET 4 | SET 5 | SET 6 |
|---|---|---|---|---|---|---|---|
| | WEIGHT | | | | | | |
| | REPS | | | | | | |
| | WEIGHT | | | | | | |
| | REPS | | | | | | |
| | WEIGHT | | | | | | |
| | REPS | | | | | | |
| | WEIGHT | | | | | | |
| | REPS | | | | | | |
| | WEIGHT | | | | | | |
| | REPS | | | | | | |
| | WEIGHT | | | | | | |
| | REPS | | | | | | |
| | WEIGHT | | | | | | |
| | REPS | | | | | | |
| | WEIGHT | | | | | | |
| | REPS | | | | | | |
| | WEIGHT | | | | | | |
| | REPS | | | | | | |
| | WEIGHT | | | | | | |
| | REPS | | | | | | |
| | WEIGHT | | | | | | |
| | REPS | | | | | | |

**CARDIO ACTIVITY:**

**NOTES:**

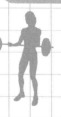

## TIP
When a craving hits don't indulge. Re-program your brain by making a cup of tea instead or going for a walk.

# YOUR TRAINING JOURNAL

**DATE**

| EXERCISE | | SET 1 | SET 2 | SET 3 | SET 4 | SET 5 | SET 6 |
|---|---|---|---|---|---|---|---|
| | WEIGHT | | | | | | |
| | REPS | | | | | | |
| | WEIGHT | | | | | | |
| | REPS | | | | | | |
| | WEIGHT | | | | | | |
| | REPS | | | | | | |
| | WEIGHT | | | | | | |
| | REPS | | | | | | |
| | WEIGHT | | | | | | |
| | REPS | | | | | | |
| | WEIGHT | | | | | | |
| | REPS | | | | | | |
| | WEIGHT | | | | | | |
| | REPS | | | | | | |
| | WEIGHT | | | | | | |
| | REPS | | | | | | |
| | WEIGHT | | | | | | |
| | REPS | | | | | | |
| | WEIGHT | | | | | | |
| | REPS | | | | | | |
| | WEIGHT | | | | | | |
| | REPS | | | | | | |

**CARDIO ACTIVITY:**

**NOTES:**

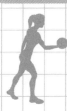

**TIP**

Enjoy yourself! You are totally on your way to a fabulous new you.

# CONTRIBUTING PHOTOGRAPHERS

Paul Buceta

Terry Goodlad

Robert Kennedy

Robert Reiff

Corey Sorenson

Stewart Volland